CHOLESTEROL AND HEART HEALTH

WHAT THE DRUG COMPANIES WON'T TELL YOU AND YOUR DOCTOR DOESN'T KNOW

THE NATURAL SOLUTIONS THAT CAN CHANGE YOUR LIFE

MICHAEL T. MURRAY, ND

18 Hueb W, Soares PR, Gersh BJ, et al. The medicine, angioplasty, or surgery study (MASS-II): a randomized, controlled clinical trial of three therapeutic strategies for multivessel coronary artery disease: one-year results. *J Am Coll Cardiol.* 2004;43(10):1743-51.

19 Graboys TB, Headley A, Lown B, et al. Results of a second-opinion program for coronary artery bypass surgery. *JAMA.* 1987;258(12):1611-4.

20 Alderman EL, Bourassa MG, Cohen LS, et al. Ten-year follow-up of survival and myocardial infarction in the randomized Coronary Artery Surgery Study. *Circulation* 1990;82(5):1629-46.

21 CASS Principal Investigators and Associates. Myocardial infarction and mortality in the Coronary Artery Surgery Study (CASS) randomized trial. *N Engl J Med.* 1984;310(12):750-8.

22 White CW, Wright CB, Doty DB, et al. Does visual interpretation of the coronary angiogram predict the physiologic importance of a coronary stenosis? *N Engl J Med.* 1984;310(13):819-24.

23 Winslow CM, Kosecoff JB, Chassin M, et al. The appropriateness of performing coronary artery bypass surgery. *JAMA.* 1988;260(4):505-9.

24 Boden WE, O'Rourke RA, Teo KK, et al. Impact of optimal medical therapy with or without percutaneous coronary intervention on long-term cardiovascular end points in patients with stable coronary artery disease (from the COURAGE Trial). *Am J Cardiol.* 2009 Jul 1;104(1):1-4.

25 Ballmer PE, Reinhart WH, Jordan P, et al. Depletion of plasma vitamin C but not vitamin E in response to cardiac operations. *J Thorac Cardiovasc Surg.* 1994;108(2):311-20.

26 Chello M, Mastroroberto P, Romano R, et al. Protection of coenzyme Q_{10} from myocardial reperfusion injury during coronary artery bypass grafting. *Ann Thorac Surg.* 1994;58(5):1427-32.

27 Clarke CN, Clarke NE, Mosher RE. Treatment of angina pectoris with disodium ethylene diamine tetraacetic acid. *Am J Med Sci.* 1956;232(6):654-66.

28 Clarke NE Sr. Atherosclerosis, occlusive vascular disease and EDTA. *Am J Cardiol.* 1960;6:233-6.

29 Steinberg D, Parthasarathy S, Carew TE, et al. Beyond cholesterol. Modifications of low-density lipoprotein that increase its atherogenicity. *N Engl J Med.* 1989;320(14):915-24.

30 Cranton EM, Frackelton JP. Current status of EDTA chelation therapy in occlusive arterial disease. *J Adv Med.* 1989;2:107-19.

31 Olszewer E, Carter JP. EDTA chelation therapy. A retrospective study of 2,870 patients. *J Adv Med.* 1989;2:197-11.

32 Olszewer E, Sabbag FC, Carter JP. A pilot double-blind study of sodium-magnesium EDTA in peripheral vascular disease. *J Natl Med Assoc.* 1990;82(3):173-7.

33 Olszewer E, Carter JP. EDTA chelation therapy in chronic degenerative disease. *Med Hypotheses.* 1988;27(1):41-9.

34 Casdorph HR. EDTA chelation therapy, efficacy in arteriosclerotic heart disease. *J Holistic Med.* 1981;3:53-9.

35 Callaway E. Chelation-therapy heart trial draws fire. *Nature.* 2012;491(7424):313-5.

36 Kidd PM. Integrated brain restoration after ischemic stroke—medical management, risk factors, nutrients, and other interventions for managing inflammation and enhancing brain plasticity. *Altern Med Rev.* 2009 Mar;14(1):14-35.

37 Aguglia E, Ban TA, Panzarasa RM, et al. Choline alphoscerate in the treatment of mental pathology following acute cerebrovascular accident. *Funct Neurol.* 1993;8:S5-S24.

38   Barbagallo Sangiorgi G, Barbagallo M, Giordano M, et al. Alpha-Glycerophosphocholine in the mental recovery of cerebral ischemic attacks. An Italian multicenter clinical trial. *Ann N Y Acad Sci.* 1994;717:253-69.

39   Consoli D, Giunta V, Grillo G, et al. [alpha-GPC in the treatment of acute cerebrovascular accident patients]. *Arch Med Interna.* 1993;45:13-23. [Article in Italian]

40   Gambi D, Onofrj M. Multicenter clinical study of efficacy and tolerability of choline alfoscerate in patients with deficits in higher mental function arising after an acute ischemic cerebrovascular attack. *Geriatria.* 1994;6:91-8.

41   Tomasina C, Manzino M, Novello P, et al. Clinical study of the therapeutic effectiveness and tolerability of choline alfoscerate in 15 subjects with compromised cognitive functions subsequent to acute focal cerebral ischemia. *Riv Neuropsichiatr Sci Affin.* 1996;37:21-8.

CHOLESTEROL AND HEART HEALTH
WHAT THE DRUG COMPANIES WON'T TELL YOU AND YOUR DOCTOR DOESN'T KNOW

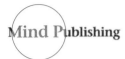

Our focus is education

COPYRIGHT © 2013 MICHAEL T. MURRAY, ND

FOR INFORMATION CONTACT

Mind Publishing Inc.
PO Box 57559,
1031 Brunette Avenue
Coquitlam, BC Canada V3K 1E0
Tel: 604-777-4330 Toll free: 1-877-477-4904
Fax: 1-866-367-5508
Email: info@mindpublishing.com
www.mindpublishing.com

ISBN: 978-1-927017-11-1
Printed in Canada

Design: FWH Creative
Editor: Donna Dawson

TABLE OF CONTENTS

ACKNOWLEDGMENTS

To my wife, Gina, for being the answer to so many of my dreams.

To my children, Lexi, Zach, and Addison, for being so incredibly magnificent and for teaching me so much about life.

To Roland Gahler and everyone at Natural Factors for their tremendous friendship and support over the years.

And finally, I am eternally grateful to all the researchers, physicians, and scientists who over the years have strived to better understand the use of natural medicines.

PREFACE

There is a lot of very good news in this book. Foremost is that heart disease can be prevented, cholesterol levels reduced, and normal blood pressure achieved through safe, effective, clinically proven natural methods – diet, lifestyle, attitude, and proper supplementation. While this book provides many answers for various heart and vascular conditions, it is not intended as a substitute for appropriate medical care. Please keep the following in mind as you read:

- **DO NOT SELF-DIAGNOSE.** If you have concerns about any subject discussed in this book, please consult a physician, preferably a naturopathic doctor (ND), nutrition-oriented medical doctor (MD), doctor of osteopathy (DO), chiropractor (DC), or other natural health care specialist. Go to naturopathic.org to find an ND in your area.

- **MAKE YOUR PHYSICIAN AWARE** of all the nutritional supplements or herbal products you are currently taking to avoid any negative interactions with any drugs you are taking.

- **IF YOU ARE CURRENTLY TAKING A PRESCRIPTION MEDICATION,** you absolutely must work with your doctor before discontinuing any drug or altering any drug regimen.

- **MOST HEALTH CONDITIONS REQUIRE A MULTIFACTORIAL SOLUTION:** medical, nutritional, and lifestyle changes. Do not rely solely on a single area of focus. You can't just take pills and not change your diet, or do the diet and the pills but ignore other lifestyle issues. Any truly effective approach to health must be truly integrated.

With the above in mind, remember that the information in this book is to be applied, not simply read. Commit yourself to following the guidelines of natural health care as detailed in this book and I believe you will be rewarded immensely

Michael T. Murray, ND
March 2013

CHAPTER 1

THE HEART OF THE MATTER IS THE MATTER OF THE HEART

Every second of every minute of your life, your heart is going to beat. The force of this vital pump pushes blood, carrying its payload of oxygen and nutrients, to every one of your tissues and organs and the cells that comprise them. Ultimately, the blood returns to the heart, where the process repeats. Each day the human heart beats about 100,000 times and pumps up to 5,000 gallons of fluid. In an average lifetime, the heart will beat 2.9 trillion times and pump 146 million gallons of blood. That's a lot of work!

The function of the heart is absolutely critical to every other part of your body – including your brain. Everything functions better when the heart works as it should. Unfortunately, millions of people operate at a deficit and are at risk of dying too soon from damage to the heart and blood vessels. Cardiovascular diseases – heart attacks and strokes – are the leading cause of death in North America and easily account for more than 30% of all deaths in the United States. Both are referred to as "silent killers" because the first symptom or sign in many cases is a fatal event.

Here's the very good news: Heart disease can be prevented. What's more, prevention doesn't require costly drugs or dangerous medical procedures. You can tune up your heart through simple but effective natural methods – diet, lifestyle, attitude, and proper supplementation.

Significant evidence shows that simply adopting a healthy diet and lifestyle dramatically reduces deaths due to cardiovascular disease (CVD). A large clinical trial enrolling over 20,000 men and women found that the combination of four healthy behaviors (not smoking, being physically active, moderate alcohol consumption, and eating at least five servings of fruit and vegetables per day) reduced total mortality fourfold compared with those who exhibited none of these behaviors.[1]

A BRIEF GUIDE TO CARDIOVASCULAR DISORDERS

The term "heart disease" is so broad that it often causes confusion. Most often doctors use the term to describe atherosclerosis (hardening of the artery walls due to a buildup of plaque containing cholesterol, fatty material, and cellular debris) of the blood vessels supplying the heart – the coronary arteries. Atherosclerosis is one main cause of heart attacks and strokes. Atherosclerosis results from the buildup of a waxy material called plaque along the walls of the blood vessel. Normally your arteries are very flexible, like a rubber tube. Plaque causes them to become stiff and can even block blood flow.

The plaque can also lead to the formation of blood clots – thickened clumps of blood that form when disk-shaped particles called platelets collect at the site of blood vessel damage. The platelets are held in place by stringy protein strands called fibrin, which is made from smaller particles called fibrinogen. Usually what happens is that the clot forms in a large vessel, where it may slow down – but not stop – blood flow. But if a piece of the clot breaks off, it will eventually circulate into a vessel that is too small to allow it to pass. As a result, blood flow to that part of the body stops, and the nearby organ or tissue can die. The bigger the clot, the bigger (and more important) the vessel it can block. The technical term for this condition is thrombosis (from the Greek word for clot.) A thromboembolism indicates that the clot has traveled away from its site of origin (*embol-* comes from the Greek meaning "to throw").

A **heart attack** (also called a myocardial infarction) occurs when something blocks the flow of blood to the heart – it can be a clot, a spasm of a coronary artery, or accumulation of plaque. Like each of your other organs, the heart needs its own supply of blood. This hard-working pump requires a steady supply of oxygen and other nutrients. The coronary arteries feed the heart. If something interrupts the blood supply, the starved muscle tissue begins to die very rapidly. The longer the blockage lasts, the greater the risk that the heart attack will be fatal.

A **stroke** is brain damage that occurs when the blood flow in the brain is interrupted or when a vessel bursts, causing blood to spurt into the surrounding tissue. While heart attacks involve coronary arteries, strokes involve arteries feeding the brain (carotid arteries). When the supply of blood is shut off, nerves in the brain die almost immediately. Sometimes the pressure of blood gushing through a ruptured vessel slices through delicate nerves, severing their millions of connections. Depending on which part of the brain is affected, damage can include loss of movement, speech, memory, or virtually any function of the body. About one third of strokes are fatal.

High blood pressure can play a critical role in the development of heart disease and strokes. In fact, it is generally regarded as the most serious risk factor for a stroke. The higher the pressure, the greater the stress on the arteries. If the vessel has a weak spot, high pressure can cause the spot to bulge or, in the case of some of the small blood vessels in the brain, possibly burst, resulting in a stroke.

Angina pectoris refers to a squeezing or pressure-like pain in the chest. It's usually caused by an insufficient supply of oxygen to the heart muscle. Angina usually precedes a heart attack. Since physical exertion and stress increase the heart's need for oxygen, they are often the triggering factors. The pain may radiate to the left shoulder blade, left arm, or jaw and typically lasts for only 1–20 minutes. Angina can be a sign of a very serious condition that needs immediate medical attention.

An **arrhythmia** is a disruption of the heart's complex pumping action. This action is governed by electrical signals. If those signals are disrupted, the chambers can start contracting in the wrong sequence. When that happens, the heart may become unable to pump enough blood to meet the body's needs.

Congestive heart failure (CHF) refers to the inability of the heart to effectively pump enough blood. Chronic CHF is most often due to long-term effects of high blood pressure, previous heart attack, disorder of a heart valve or the heart muscle, or chronic lung diseases such as asthma or emphysema. Weakness, fatigue, and shortness of breath are the most common symptoms of CHF.

UNDERSTANDING ATHEROSCLEROSIS

To fully understand the important ways that the various natural measures described in this chapter affect the health of the arteries and the treatment of CVD, it is necessary to closely examine the structure of an artery and the process of atherosclerosis.

STRUCTURE OF AN ARTERY

An artery is divided into three major layers:

1. The intima is the internal lining of the artery (the medical term is "endothelium"). The intima consists of a layer of cells known as endothelial cells. Molecules known as glycosaminoglycans (GAGs) line the exposed

endothelial cells to protect them from damage and to promote repair. Beneath the surface endothelial cells is the internal elastic membrane, composed of a layer of GAGs and other compounds, which supports the endothelial cells and separates the intima from the smooth muscle layer.

2. The media, or middle layer, consists primarily of smooth muscle cells. Interspersed among the cells are GAGs and other structures, which provide support and elasticity to the artery.

3. The adventitia, or external elastic membrane, consists primarily of connective tissue, including GAGs, providing structural support and elasticity to the artery.

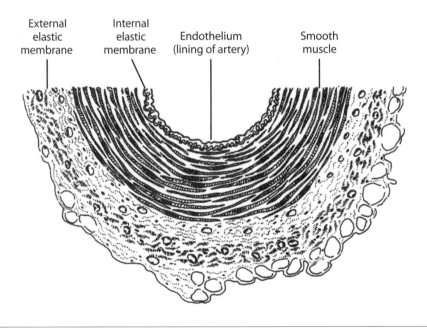

Figure 1.1 Structure of an Artery

THE PROCESS OF ATHEROSCLEROSIS

No single theory of the development of atherosclerosis satisfies all investigators. The most widely accepted explanation theorizes that the lesions of atherosclerosis are initiated as a response to injury to the cells lining the inside of the artery, the arterial endothelium. Details of the progression of atherosclerosis are illustrated in Figure 1.2.

Atherosclerosis begins when something happens to damage the GAG layer that protects the inner lining of the blood vessel. That "something" might be the presence of a pathogen, such as a virus; a drug or environmental toxin; physical damage due to a spasm or high blood pressure; or an over-eager immune response.

Like a leak in a dike, even a small amount of damage to the inner lining can set a deadly chain of events in motion. One critical thing that happens is that fat-carrying proteins (lipoproteins), always circulating in the blood, start attaching themselves to the GAGs, like unwanted bystanders at a traffic accident. The low-density lipoproteins (LDL) carry cholesterol away from the liver. Thus, their arrival causes cholesterol to build up. When LDL binds to the site, it begins to break down, or oxidize. This releases free radicals, which further damage nearby cells. This mechanism is why dietary cholesterol is such a major risk factor for heart disease. The more you have in your blood, the more it can pile up at the site of damage to the blood vessel.

Vessel damage sets off alarms, spurring your body's repair mechanism into action. The damaged cells secrete growth factors that stimulate cells to reproduce and replace damaged cells. The cells also release fibrinogen, the sticky, stringy protein that collects platelets so a clot can form to prevent blood from leaking out of the vessel. White blood cells, ever helpful, arrive at the site and attach themselves to the vessel wall, turning into macrophages. These cells are on duty to destroy any harmful particles, such as oxidized LDLs. But once they become stuffed with LDL, they change into useless blobs called foam cells and lose their scavenging ability.

Macrophages also contribute their own supply of growth factor. All this growth factor causes cells from the smooth muscle layer of the vessel to start migrating toward the inner layer. Once there, they begin replicating. In the process these cells dump cellular debris, such as fiber-like proteins, into the intima, adding more trash to the heap. Soon a kind of scar tissue, called a fibrous cap, appears on the surface of the artery lining. This combination of lipoprotein, cholesterol, fibrous protein, and biological litter forms a stiff patch called atherosclerotic plaque. Over time the plaque continues to grow until eventually it blocks the entire artery.

Your blood flow can be reduced by up to 90% before you feel any symptoms of atherosclerosis. By then it may be too late. You are a heart attack waiting to happen.

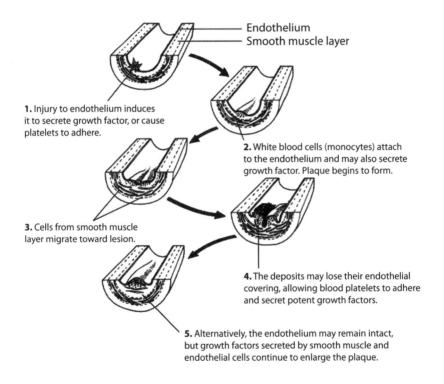

Figure 1.2 Development of Atherosclerosis

CAUSES

Prevention of atherosclerosis and CVD involves reducing and, when possible, eliminating various risk factors. Risk factors are divided into two primary categories: major risk factors and other risk factors (Table 1.1). Keep in mind that some of the "other" risk factors have actually been shown to be more important than the so-called major risk factors. For example, a strong argument could be made that insulin resistance and elevations in high-sensitivity C-reactive protein (hsCRP), a marker for inflammation, are much more important than elevated cholesterol levels. It is also important to point out that the risk for a heart attack increases exponentially with the number of risk factors a person has (see Table 1.2).

Table 1.1 Risk Factors for Atherosclerosis

Major Risk Factors	Other Risk Factors
Smoking	Elevations of high-sensitivity C-reactive protein
Elevated blood cholesterol levels (especially oxidized LDL, known as oxLDL)	Insulin resistance
High blood pressure	Low thyroid function
Diabetes	Low antioxidant status
Physical inactivity	Low levels of essential fatty acids
	Increased platelet aggregation
	Increased fibrinogen formation
	Low levels of magnesium or potassium
	Elevated levels of homocysteine
	"Type A" personality

Table 1.2 Association of Major Risk Factors with Incidence of Atherosclerosis

Major Risk Factors	% Increase in Incidence
Presence of one major risk factor	30
High cholesterol and high blood pressure	300
High cholesterol and smoking	350
High blood pressure and smoking	350
Smoking, high blood cholesterol, and high blood pressure	720

CLINICAL EVALUATION FOR CARDIOVASCULAR DISEASE

Since CVDs are such a major cause of death, I recommend consulting a physician to have a complete cardiovascular assessment, which could include the tests listed in Table 1.3. This recommendation is especially important if you have any major risk factor for atherosclerosis or a strong family history of heart disease.

Table 1.3 Assessment of the Cardiovascular System

Laboratory Tests	Other Procedures
Total cholesterol (oxLDL more predictive)	Exercise stress test
Low-density lipoprotein cholesterol	Electrocardiography
High-density lipoprotein cholesterol	Echocardiography
High-sensitivity C-reactive protein	
Lipoprotein(a)	
Fibrinogen	
Homocysteine	
Ferritin (an iron-binding protein)	
Lipid peroxides	

DETERMINING YOUR RISK

To help determine your overall risk for having a heart attack or stroke, I developed the following risk-determinant scale. Although this risk assessment does not take into consideration several other important factors – such as the level of fibrinogen and coping style – the score provides a good indication of your relative risk for a heart attack or stroke. Each of these risk factors is briefly discussed below and many will be further discussed in more detail in subsequent chapters.

Table 1.4 Risk Determination Scale for Heart Disease and Stroke

Risk Factor	Risk Scale				
	1	2	3	4	5
Blood pressure (systolic)	≤125	125–134	135–149	150–164	≥165
Blood pressure (diastolic)	≤90	90–94	95–104	105–114	≥115
Smoking (cigarettes per day)	None	1–9	10–19	20–29	≥30
Heredity I*	None	≥65	50–64	35–49	≤35
Heredity II†	0	1	2	4	≥4
Diabetes duration (years)	0	1–5	6–10	11–15	≥15
Total cholesterol (mg/dl)	≤200	200–224	225–249	250–274	≥275
HDL (mg/dl)	≥75	65–74	55–64	35–54	≤35
Total cholesterol/HDL ratio‡	≤3	3–3.9	4–4.9	5–6.4	≥6.5
High-sensitivity CRP (mg/l)	≤1	1–1.9	2–2.9	3–4	≥4
Exercise (hours per week)	≥4	3–4	2–3	1–2	≤1
Supplemental EPA/DHA intake (mg)	≥600	400–599	200–399	100–199	≤100
Vitamin C, vitamin E, selenium, PCO source, lutein supplementation (number of items)	5	3	2	1	0
Average daily servings of fruit and vegetables	≥5	4–5	3	1–2	0
Age	≤35	36–45	46–55	56–65	≥65
TOTALS					

HDL = high-density lipoprotein cholesterol; **CRP** = C-reactive protein;
EPA = eicosapentaenoic acid; **DHA** = docosahexaenoic acid;
PCO = procyanidolic oligomer.

*Age of patient when he or she had a heart attack or stroke.

†Number of immediate family members having had a heart attack before age 50.

‡Total cholesterol value is divided by HDL value.

Risk = sum of all five columns:
14–20 = very low; 21–30 = low; 31–40 = average; 41–50 = high; ≥51 = very high.

EARLOBE CREASE

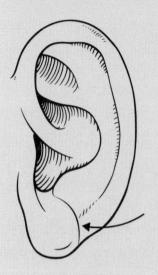

The presence of a diagonal earlobe crease has been recognized as a sign of CVD since 1973. More than 30 studies have been reported in the medical literature. The earlobe is richly vascularized, and a decrease in blood flow over an extended period is believed to result in collapse of the vascular bed. This leads to a diagonal crease.[2,3]

Figure 1.3 Diagonal Earlobe Crease

In one study, angiographs performed on 205 consecutive patients showed an 82% accuracy in predicting heart disease, with a false positive rate of 12% and a false negative rate of 18%. In another study of 112 consecutive patients, the earlobe crease was highly correlated with demonstrable heart disease and less strongly with a previous heart attack.[2]

The crease is seen more commonly with advancing age, until the age of 80, when the incidence drops dramatically. However, the association with heart disease is independent of age. Although the presence of an earlobe crease does not prove heart disease, it strongly suggests it, and examination of the earlobe is an easy screening procedure. The correlation does not hold with Asians or Native Americans.[3]

A QUICK LOOK AT RISK FACTORS

SMOKING

Cigarette smoking is perhaps the most important risk factor for atherosclerosis and CVD: Statistical evidence reveals that smokers have a 70% greater risk of death from CVD than nonsmokers do.[4] The more cigarettes smoked and the more years a person has smoked, the greater the risk of dying from a heart attack or stroke. Overall, the average smoker dies 7–8 years sooner than the average nonsmoker.

Tobacco smoke contains more than 4,000 chemicals, of which more than 50 have been identified as carcinogens. These chemicals are extremely damaging to the cardiovascular system. Specifically, they are carried in the bloodstream on low-density lipoprotein cholesterol (LDL; the "bad" cholesterol), where they either damage the lining of the arteries directly or they damage the LDL molecule (creating oxidized LDL), which then damages the arteries. An elevated LDL level worsens the effect of smoking on the cardiovascular system because more cigarette toxins travel through it.

Smoking contributes to elevated cholesterol presumably by damaging feedback mechanisms in the liver, which control how much cholesterol the liver manufactures.[3] Smoking also promotes the formation of blood clots because it increases both platelet aggregation and blood fibrinogen levels, two other important independent risk factors for CVD. In addition, it is a well-documented fact that cigarette smoking contributes to high blood pressure.[5]

Even passive exposure to cigarette smoke is damaging to cardiovascular health: Convincing evidence links environmental (secondhand or passive) smoke to CVD. Analysis of 10 population-based studies indicates a consistent dose-response effect related to exposure.[6] In other words, the more you are exposed to cigarette smoke the greater your risk for CVD. Evidence indicates that nonsmokers appear to be more sensitive to smoke, including its negative effects on the cardiovascular system.

Environmental tobacco smoke actually has a higher concentration of some toxic constituents than the smoke that smokers inhale. Data collected after short- and long-term environmental tobacco smoke exposure shows changes in the lining of the arteries and in platelet function as well as exercise capacity similar to those in active smoking. In summary, passive smoking is a relevant risk factor for CVD. In the United States it is estimated that more than 37,000 coronary heart disease (CHD) deaths each year are attributable to environmental smoke.

The good news is that the magnitude of risk reduction achieved by quitting smoking in patients with CVD is quite significant. Results from a detailed meta-analysis showed a 36% reduction in relative risk of mortality for patients with coronary artery disease who quit compared with those who continued smoking.[7]

Various measures – including nicotine skin patches or chewing gum, acupuncture, and hypnosis – have all been shown to provide some benefit in helping patients quit smoking, but not much. A systematic review of the efficacy of interventions intended to help people to stop smoking analyzed data from 188 randomized controlled trials.[8] Encouragement to stop smoking by physicians during a routine office call resulted in a 2% cessation rate after one year. Supplementary measures such as follow-up letters or visits had an additional effect. Behavioral modification techniques such as relaxation, rewards and punishments, and avoiding trigger situations in group or individual sessions led by a psychologist had no greater effect than the 2% rate achieved by simple advice from a physician. Eight studies with acupuncture have produced an overall effectiveness rate of roughly 3%. Hypnosis has been judged to be ineffective even though trials have shown a success rate of 23%. Hypnosis was judged to be ineffective because no biochemical marker was used to accurately determine effectiveness. Nicotine replacement therapy (gum or patch) is effective in about 13% of smokers who seek help in quitting. All together, these results are not encouraging. It appears that the best results occur when people quit "cold turkey."

TIPS TO **STOP SMOKING**

1. List all the reasons you want to quit smoking and review them daily.

2. Set a specific day to quit, tell at least 10 friends that you are going to quit smoking, and then DO IT!

3. Throw away all cigarettes, butts, matches, and ash trays.

4. Use substitutes. Instead of smoking, chew on raw vegetables, fruit, or gum. If your fingers seem empty, play with a pencil.

5. Take one day at a time.

6. Realize that 40 million Americans have quit. If they can do it, so can you!

7. Visualize yourself as a nonsmoker with a fatter pocketbook, pleasant breath, unstained teeth, and the satisfaction that comes from being in control of your life.

8. Join an Internet support group. While the research is early, it appears that doing so can double or even triple success rates.

9. When you need to relax, perform deep breathing exercises rather than reaching for a cigarette.

10. Avoid situations that you associate with smoking.

11. Each day, reward yourself in a positive way. Buy yourself something with the money you've saved or plan a special reward as a celebration for quitting.

ELEVATED BLOOD CHOLESTEROL LEVELS

The evidence overwhelmingly demonstrates that elevated cholesterol levels greatly increase the risk of death due to CVD, especially elevations in LDL cholesterol.[8] It's currently recommended that the total blood cholesterol level be less than 200 mg/dl. In addition, it is recommended that the LDL be less than 130 mg/dl, the high-density lipoprotein cholesterol (HDL; "good" cholesterol) greater than 35 mg/dl, and the triglyceride level less than 150 mg/dl.

Cholesterol is transported in the blood by lipoproteins. The major categories of lipoproteins are very-low-density lipoprotein (VLDL), LDL, and HDL. Because VLDL and LDL are responsible for transporting fats (primarily triglycerides and cholesterol) from the liver to body cells, while HDL is responsible for returning fats to the liver, elevations of either VLDL or LDL are associated with an increased risk for developing atherosclerosis, the primary cause of heart attacks and strokes. In contrast, elevations of HDL are associated with a lower risk of heart attacks.

The ratios of total cholesterol to HDL cholesterol and LDL to HDL are referred to as the cardiac risk factor ratios because they reflect whether cholesterol is being deposited into tissues or broken down and excreted. The ratio of total cholesterol to HDL should be no higher than 4.2, and the LDL:HDL ratio should be no higher than 2.5. The risk of heart disease can be reduced dramatically by lowering LDL while simultaneously raising HDL levels: For every 1% drop in the LDL level, the risk of a heart attack drops by 2%. Conversely, for every 1% increase in HDL level, the risk for a heart attack drops 3–4%.[9,10]

Lowering total cholesterol, LDL, and triglycerides, and increasing HDL, are clearly associated with reducing CVD risk. Strategies for accomplishing these goals are given in Chapter 3, The Truth About Statins, Cholesterol, and Natural Alternatives.

DIABETES

Atherosclerosis is one of the key underlying factors in the development of many chronic complications of diabetes. Individuals with diabetes have a twofold to threefold higher risk of dying prematurely of heart disease or stroke than those who are not diabetic, and 55% of deaths in diabetic patients are caused by CVD. However, even mild insulin resistance and poor glucose control have both been shown to dramatically affect the incidence and progression of CVD. The role of diabetes and insulin resistance is discussed in more detail below and in Chapter 4, Beyond Cholesterol: The Role of Insulin Resistance.

HIGH BLOOD PRESSURE

Elevated blood pressure is often a sign of considerable atherosclerosis and is a major risk factor for heart attack or stroke. In fact, the presence of high blood pressure is generally regarded as the most significant risk factor for stroke. Strategies to lower blood pressure are given in Chapter 6, High Blood Pressure.

PHYSICAL INACTIVITY

A sedentary lifestyle is another major risk factor for CVD. "Physical activity" refers to "bodily movement produced by skeletal muscles that requires energy expenditure" and produces health benefits. Exercise, a type of physical activity, is defined as "planned, structured, and repetitive bodily movement done to improve or maintain one or more components of physical fitness." Physical inactivity denotes a level of activity less than that needed to maintain good health. It applies to most Americans, as roughly 54% of adults report little or no regular physical activity; there has also been a sharp decline in regular exercise among children and adolescents.[11]

Physical activity and regular exercise protect against the development of CVD and also favorably modify other CVD risk factors, including high blood pressure, blood lipid levels, insulin resistance, and obesity. Exercise is also important in the treatment and management of patients who have CVD or are at increased risk, including those who have high blood pressure, stable angina, a prior heart attack, peripheral vascular disease, or heart failure, or who are recovering from a cardiovascular event. For more information, see Chapter 5, The Heart Healthy Lifestyle.

OTHER RISK FACTORS

In addition to the major risk factors for CVD described above, a number of other factors have, on occasion, been shown to be more significant than the so-called major risk factors. In fact, more than 300 different risk factors have

RELIGION AND THE HEART

Researcher Jeff Levin, PhD, author of *God, Faith and Health,* is recognized
as one of the leading researchers in the field of spirituality and health. As a
first-year graduate student in the School of Public Health at the University of
North Carolina in Chapel Hill, Levin became intrigued by two articles that found
a surprising and significant connection between spirituality and heart disease, a
connection that remains one of the best-researched areas of the positive effects
of religious behavior on health. His curiosity led to an in-depth evaluation and
pioneering research on the impact of religious practices on disease.

In *God, Faith and Health,* Dr. Levin notes that in more than 50 studies, religious
practices were found to protect against heart disease, including death due to heart
attacks and strokes, as well as the incidence of numerous risk factors, including
high blood pressure and elevated cholesterol and triglyceride levels. In particular,
Dr. Levin highlights the strong inverse correlation between strong religious commitment and blood pressure that was evident no matter what religion an individual
chose to practice or his or her geographical location or ancestry.

been identified. Although there is considerable evidence that all of these risk
factors and more can play significant roles in the progression of atherosclerosis, much of the current research has focused on the central roles of inflammatory processes, insulin resistance, platelet aggregation, and fibrinogen.

SILENT INFLAMMATION

Inflammation is a reaction designed to protect us after an injury or infection. The term owes its origin to the Latin word *inflammare,* which means
to set on fire. In the classic response to injury or infection, the injured area
becomes red, swollen, hot, and painful. But there is another type of inflam-

mation that is not so obvious. This silent inflammation reflects an underlying low-grade stimulation of the inflammatory process with no outward signs of inflammation. The only way it is apparent is by looking at blood for markers of inflammation, such as C-reactive protein (discussed in detail below). Silent inflammation is a major factor in the development of virtually every major chronic degenerative disease, including CVD, type 2 diabetes, cancer, and Alzheimer's disease.

Many factors trigger silent inflammation, including resistance to the hormone insulin, obesity, emotional stress, environmental toxins, low antioxidant intake or increased exposure to free radicals (e.g., from radiation or smoking), chronic infections, imbalances of dietary fats, and increased intestinal permeability.

Inflammatory mediators influence many stages in the development of atherosclerosis, from initial leukocyte recruitment to eventual rupture of unstable atherosclerotic plaque. In particular, high-sensitivity C-reactive protein, a blood marker that reflects different degrees of inflammation, has been identified as an independent risk factor for CAD. Although the hsCRP level has been shown to be a stronger predictor of cardiovascular events than the LDL level, screening for both biological markers provides a better prediction than screening for either alone.[12]

Elevations in hsCRP are closely linked to insulin resistance, which means cells of the body become unresponsive to the hormone insulin (see Chapter 4, Beyond Cholesterol: The Role of Insulin Resistance).[13] Insulin resistance is a key underlying factor not only in type 2 diabetes, but also in metabolic syndrome, defined as a combination of at least three of the following metabolic risk factors:

- Central obesity (a waist-to-hip ratio greater than 1 for men and greater than 0.8 for women)

- Blood triglycerides greater than 150 mg/dl and low HDL (below 40 mg/dl in men and below 50 mg/dl in women)

- High blood pressure (130/85 mm Hg or higher)

- Insulin resistance or glucose intolerance (fasting blood sugar levels above 101 mg/dl)

- Prothrombotic state (e.g., high fibrinogen or plasminogen activator inhibitor in the blood)

- Pro-inflammatory state (e.g., elevated hsCRP in the blood)

Metabolic syndrome has become increasingly common in the United States. It is now estimated that more than 60 million U.S. adults may have it. Insulin resistance and metabolic syndrome are closely tied to obesity (particularly abdominal obesity), elevations in hsCRP, and a significant risk for CAD. Strategies for dealing with insulin resistance and diabetes are discussed fully in Chapter 4, Beyond Cholesterol: The Role of Insulin Resistance.

PLATELET AGGREGATION

Excessive platelet aggregation is another independent risk factor for heart disease and stroke. Once platelets aggregate, they release potent compounds that dramatically promote the formation of atherosclerotic plaque. They can also form a clot that can lodge in small arteries and produce a heart attack or stroke. The adhesiveness of platelets is determined largely by the type of fats in the diet and the level of antioxidants. While saturated fats and cholesterol increase platelet aggregation, omega-3 oils (both short-chain and long-chain) and monounsaturated fats have the opposite effect. The role of dietary fats as well as antioxidant nutrients and flavonoids is discussed in detail in the next chapter. In addition to these factors, vitamin B6 also inhibits platelet aggregation and lowers blood pressure and homocysteine levels.[14,15]

One study determined the effect of vitamin B6 (pyridoxine hydrochloride) supplementation on platelet aggregation, cholesterol, and serum zinc levels in 24 healthy male volunteers (19–24 years old) given either B6 at a dosage of 5 mg/kg body weight or a placebo for four weeks.[14] Results demonstrated that pyridoxine inhibited platelet aggregation by 41–48%, while there was no change in the control group. Vitamin B6 was also shown to lower total cholesterol levels considerably from pretreatment levels. Total cholesterol was reduced from 156 to 116 mg/dl. HDL increased from 37.9 to 48.6 mg/dl.

Another study showed the blood level of the active form of vitamin B_6 – pyridoxal-5-phosphate (P5P) – to be inversely related to both hsCRP and fibrinogen.[15] In other words, the lower the level of P5P, the higher the level of hsCRP. Low P5P concentrations were associated with a calculated 89% increased risk for CVD.

Non-antioxidant vitamins and minerals may also be important in support-ing the effectiveness of antioxidants. Taking a multivitamin/multimineral supplement rather than simply taking vitamin B_6 seems to make the most sense. In one double-blind study, hsCRP levels were significantly lower in a group taking a multivitamin than in a placebo group. The reduction in hsCRP levels was most evident in patients who had elevated levels (1 mg/l or more) at baseline.[16] Researchers found that serum vitamin B_6 and vita-min C levels were inversely associated with the hsCRP level. The results from all these studies provide clear evidence of the possible role of vitamin B6 supplementation in reducing the risk of CVD mortality.

Garlic preparations standardized for alliin content, as well as garlic oil, have also demonstrated inhibition of platelet aggregation. In one study, 120 patients with increased platelet aggregation were given either 900 mg/day of a dried garlic preparation containing 1.3% alliin or a placebo for four weeks.[17] In the garlic group, spontaneous platelet aggregation disappeared, the microcirculation of the skin increased by 47.6%, plasma viscosity de-creased by 3.2%, diastolic blood pressure dropped from an average of 74 to 67 mm Hg, and fasting blood glucose concentration dropped from an average of 89.4 to 79 mg/dl.

FIBRINOGEN

Fibrinogen is a component of blood clots and atherosclerotic plaque. Ele-vated fibrinogen levels are another clear risk factor for CVD. Early clinical studies stimulated detailed population-based investigations into the possible link between fibrinogen and CVD. The first such study was the Northwick Park Heart Study in the United Kingdom. This large study involved 1,510 men 40–64 years of age who were randomly recruited and tested for a range of clotting factors, including fibrinogen. At the four-year follow-up, there was a stronger association between cardiovascular deaths and fibrinogen levels than for cholesterol. This association has now been confirmed in at least five other large population-based studies.[18]

Natural therapies designed to promote fibrinolysis include exercise, omega-3 oils, niacin, garlic, and nattokinase. In addition, the Mediterranean diet alone significantly reduces fibrinogen and other markers of inflammation.[19] This diet is described in detail in Chapter 2, Basic Dietary and Supplement Strategies for Heart Health. Adherence to the Mediterranean diet was shown to be associated with a 20% lower CRP level, 17% lower interleukin-6 level, 15% lower homocysteine level, and 6% lower fibrinogen level.

Natto is a traditional Japanese food prepared from soybeans fermented with Bacillus subtilis. Nattokinase is a protein-digesting enzyme isolated from natto; it has potent fibrinolytic and thrombolytic ("clot-busting") activity that has shown significant potential in improving CVD.[20] Specifically, nattokinase has been shown to:

- Dissolve excess fibrin in blood vessels, which improves circulation, causes clot dissolution, and reduces risk of severe clotting to prevent strokes and heart attacks

- Reduce LDL (bad) cholesterol and increases HDL (good) cholesterol

- Reduce blood viscosity, improves blood flow, and lowers blood pressure

The ability to improve blood vessel health was quite obvious in a double-blind study in patients with high blood pressure.[21] In the study, 73 subjects with baseline untreated moderate high blood pressure of 130–159/100–120 mm Hg were randomized to take either nattokinase (2000 FU/capsule per day) or placebo. After eight weeks, subjects in the nattokinase group showed a significant reduction in systolic blood pressure (5.5 mm Hg) and diastolic blood pressure (2.84 mm Hg), compared with subjects in the placebo group. The typical dosage for nattokinase is 100 mg (2000 FU) once or twice daily.

HOMOCYSTEINE

Homocysteine is an intermediate in the conversion of the amino acid methionine to cysteine that can damage the lining of arteries, as well as the brain. If a person is functionally deficient in folic acid, vitamin B_6, or vitamin B_{12}, there will be an increase in homocysteine. Elevated homocysteine levels are an independent risk factor for heart attack, stroke, and peripheral vascular disease. Elevations in homocysteine are found in approximately 20–40% of patients with heart disease and are significantly associated with CVD.[22–25]

Although folic acid supplementation (400 mcg daily) alone can reduce homocysteine levels in many people, given the importance of vitamins B_6 and B_{12} to proper homocysteine metabolism, all three should be used together. In one study the suboptimal levels of these nutrients in men with elevated homocysteine levels were 56.8% for folic acid, 59.1% for vitamin B_{12}, and 25% for vitamin B_6, indicating that folic acid supplementation alone would not lower homocysteine levels in many cases.[26] In other words, folic acid supplementation will lower homocysteine levels only if there are adequate levels of vitamins B_6 and B_{12}.

In 1998 the Food and Drug Administration mandated the fortification of some food products with folic acid. Although homocysteine levels have decreased modestly since then, the effect on mortality has been minor at best.[27] This indicates the importance of supplementing all three nutrients, not just one.

"TYPE A" PERSONALITY

"Type A" behavior is characterized by an extreme sense of time urgency, competitiveness, impatience, and aggression. This behavior carries with it a twofold increase in CHD compared with non-type A behavior.[28–30] Particularly damaging to the cardiovascular system is the regular expression of anger. In one study, the relationship between habitual anger coping styles, especially anger expression, and serum lipid concentrations were examined in 86 healthy people.[29] Habitual anger expression was measured on four scales: aggression, controlled affect (mood), guilt, and social inhibition. A positive correlation between serum cholesterol level and aggression was found: The higher the aggression score, the higher the cholesterol level. A negative correlation was found between the LDL:HDL ratio and the controlled affect score – the greater the ability to control anger, the lower this ratio.

In other words, those who learn to control anger experience a significant reduction in the risk for heart disease, while an unfavorable lipid profile is linked with a predominantly aggressive (hostile) anger coping style.

Anger expression also plays a role in CRP levels. In one study, greater anger and severity of depressive symptoms, separately and in combination with hostility, were significantly associated with elevations in CRP in apparently healthy men and women.[30] Other mechanisms explaining the link between the emotions, personality, and CVD include increased cortisol secretion, endothelial dysfunction, high blood pressure, and increased platelet aggregation and fibrinogen levels.[31]

FINAL COMMENTS

One of the most popular recommendations given by physicians for reducing the risk of a heart attack is to take low-dose aspirin (e.g., less than 325 mg/day). While aspirin has been shown to decrease the risk of heart attacks and strokes both in people who have not had a heart attack (primary prevention) and those with a history of a heart attack (secondary prevention), it may not be the best approach.

The best approach to preventing first or subsequent heart attacks may be one that is too often overlooked by many physicians – diet. Several studies have shown that dietary modifications are not only more effective in preventing recurrent heart attack than aspirin but can also reverse the blockage of clogged arteries.[32–34] The benefits of the important dietary and supplement strategies given in Chapter 2 far exceed any possible benefit from the simplistic recommendation of taking aspirin to prevent a heart attack.

There is also some risk of ulcer formation with aspirin use, even at low dosages. The risk of gastrointestinal bleeding due to peptic ulcers has been evaluated for aspirin at daily dosages of 300, 150, and 75 mg. Essentially, there is an increased risk of gastrointestinal bleeding due to peptic ulcers at all dosage levels. However, the dosage of 75 mg/day was associated with a 2.3-fold increased risk of ulcers, compared with a 3.2-fold increased risk at 150 mg/day and a 3.9-fold increased risk at 300 mg/day.[35]

It is important to point out that there are only positive side effects with the use of dietary, lifestyle, and proven supplement strategies to reduce heart attack and stroke risk. When additional factors that affect platelet aggregation are considered, such as fish oils, garlic and onions, and special factors such as nattokinase, there is little doubt that a natural approach can be constructed that goes well beyond the small benefit that aspirin may produce.

CHAPTER 2

BASIC DIETARY AND SUPPLEMENTAL STRATEGIES FOR HEART HEALTH

It is now well established that certain dietary practices cause heart disease, while others can prevent it. Clearly, the standard American diet contributes greatly to heart disease. It's not just that the standard American diet is too high in fat, cholesterol, fried foods, and animal protein, it's also high in sugar and other refined carbohydrates. High-sugar "junk food" diets contribute to heart disease in a major way by leading to poor blood sugar regulation, obesity, and ultimately type 2 diabetes. A study of more than 48,000 participants followed for an average of eight years found that the consumption of foods that caused a rapid rise in blood sugar levels (a high-glycemic-load diet) increased the risk of cardiovascular disease (CVD) by 68%.[1]

As for diet in the prevention of heart disease, one of the most widely studied dietary interventions in CVD is the traditional "Mediterranean diet." This diet reflects food patterns typical of some Mediterranean regions in the early 1960s, such as Crete, parts of the rest of Greece, and southern Italy. Unfortunately the modern Mediterranean diet has deviated significantly from its healthful origin. The original Mediterranean diet had the following characteristics:

- Olive oil is the principal source of fat.

- The diet centers on an abundance of plant food (fruit; potatoes, beans, and other vegetables; breads; pasta; nuts; and seeds).

- Foods are minimally processed, and people focus on seasonally fresh and locally grown foods.

- Fresh fruit is the typical daily dessert, with sweets containing concentrated sugars or honey consumed only a few times a week at most.

- Dairy products (principally cheese and yogurt) are consumed daily in low to moderate amounts.

- Fish is consumed regularly.

- Poultry and eggs are consumed in moderate amounts (up to four times weekly) or not at all.

- Red meat is consumed in low amounts.

- Wine is consumed in low to moderate amounts, normally with meals.

One study examined the effect of the Mediterranean diet on the lining of blood vessels and high-sensitivity C-reactive protein (hsCRP) in patients with metabolic syndrome.[2] Patients in the intervention group were instructed to follow the Mediterranean diet and received detailed advice on how to increase their daily consumption of whole grains, fruit, vegetables, nuts, and olive oil. Patients in the control group followed the American Heart Association (AHA) diet. After two years, patients following the Mediterranean diet consumed more foods rich in monounsaturated fat, polyunsaturated fat, and fiber and had a lower ratio of omega-6 to omega-3 fatty acids. Compared with patients consuming the AHA diet, patients consuming the Mediterranean diet had significantly reduced serum concentrations of hsCRP and other inflammatory mediators, improved blood vessel function, and greater weight loss.

Although several components of the Mediterranean diet deserve special mention, it is important to stress that the total benefits reflect an interplay among many beneficial compounds rather than any single factor.[3] Some of the key benefits of the Mediterranean diet are that it reduces silent inflammation, aids in blood sugar stability, and improves insulin sensitivity.

OLIVE OIL AND OMEGA-3 FATTY ACIDS

Another important aspect of the Mediterranean diet may be the combination of olive oil (a source of monounsaturated fats and antioxidants) and the intake of omega-3 fatty acids. Olive oil contains not only monounsaturated fatty acid (oleic acid) but also several antioxidant agents that may account for some of its health benefits. In addition to a mild effect in lowering low-density lipoprotein cholesterol (LDL; "bad" cholesterol) and triglycerides, olive oil increases high-density lipoprotein cholesterol (HDL; "good" cholesterol) and helps prevent LDL from being damaged by free radicals, creating oxidized LDL, which is even more damaging to the arteries.[4]

More than 300 clinical trials have also demonstrated the benefits of the longer-chain omega-3 fatty acids eicosapentaenoic acid (EPA) and docosahexaenoic acid (DHA) for cardiovascular health. These fatty acids exert considerable benefits on reducing the risk for CVD. Supplementation with EPA and DHA has little effect on cholesterol levels but does lower triglyceride levels significantly and produces myriad additional beneficial effects, including reduced platelet aggregation, improved function of the lining of blood vessels, improved arterial flexibility, improved blood and oxygen supply to the heart, and a mild effect in lowering blood pressure.[5]

The levels of EPA and DHA within red blood cells have been shown to be highly significant predictors of heart disease. This laboratory value has been termed the omega-3 index. An omega-3 index of 8% was associated with the greatest protection, whereas an index of 4% was associated with the least. One analysis showed the omega-3 index to be the most significant predictor of CVD, better than hsCRP; total cholesterol, LDL, or HDL; or homocysteine. Researchers subsequently determined that 1000 mg daily of EPA and DHA combined is required to achieve or surpass the 8% omega-3 index target.[6,7]

The omega-3 index findings are not surprising, as a wealth of information has documented a clear relationship between dietary consumption of omega-3 fatty acids and the likelihood of developing CVD: The higher the omega-3 fatty acid intake, the lower the likelihood of CVD. It has been estimated that raising the levels of long-chain omega-3 fatty acids through diet or supplementation may reduce overall cardiovascular mortality by as much as 45%.[8,9]

In general, for preventive effects against CVD, the dosage recommendation is 1000 mg EPA+DHA per day; for lowering triglycerides, the dosage is 3000 mg per day. In a double-blind study, after eight weeks of supplementation, a daily dosage of 3400 mg EPA+DHA lowered triglycerides by 27%, while a lower dosage of 850 mg had no effect. These results clearly indicate that the effective dosage for lowering triglycerides with fish oils is 3000 mg EPA+DHA per day.[10]

Although the longer-chain omega-3 fatty acids exert more pronounced effects than alpha-linolenic acid – the shorter-chain omega-3 fatty acid from vegetable sources (e.g., flaxseed oil, walnuts) – it is important to point out that the two populations with the lowest rates of heart attack have a relatively high intake of alpha-linolenic acid: the Japanese who inhabit Kohama Island and the inhabitants of Crete.[11,12] Typically, Cretans have a threefold higher serum concentration of alpha-linolenic acid than residents of other European countries, owing to their frequent consumption of walnuts and the vegetable purslane.[11] Of course another important dietary factor in both the Kohamans and Cretans is their use of oils containing oleic acid. However, although the oleic acid content of the diet offers some degree of protection, the rates of heart attack among the Kohamans and Cretans are much lower than those in populations that consume only oleic acid sources and little alpha-linolenic acid. The intake of alpha-linolenic acid is viewed as a more significant protective factor than oleic acid.

TAKE A HIGH-QUALITY FISH OIL SUPPLEMENT

One of the major advances in nutritional medicine is the ability to produce a fish oil supplement that is a highly concentrated form of long-chain omega-3 fatty acids and also free from lipid peroxides, heavy metals, environmental contaminants, and other harmful compounds. These "pharmaceutical grade" fish oil concentrates are so superior to earlier fish oil products that they are literally revolutionizing nutritional medicine because of the health benefits they produce.

When selecting a fish oil supplement, it is essential to use a brand that you trust. Quality control is an absolute must to ensure the product is free from heavy metals such as lead and mercury, pesticides, damaged fats (lipid peroxides), and other contaminants. For general health, the recommended dosage is 1000 mg of EPA+DHA daily. Read the label carefully – it's not 1000 mg of fish oil, it's 1000 mg of EPA+DHA that is required. For therapeutic purposes such as reducing inflammation or lowering triglyceride levels the dosage recommendation is usually 3000 mg EPA+DHA daily.

NUTS AND SEEDS

Higher consumption of nuts and seeds has been shown to significantly reduce the risk of CVD in large population-based studies.[13] Researchers estimate that substituting nuts for an equivalent amount of carbohydrates in an average diet resulted in a 30% reduction in heart disease risk. Researchers calculated an even more impressive risk reduction, 45%, when fat from nuts was substituted for saturated fats (found primarily in meat and dairy products). Nuts have a cholesterol-lowering effect, which partly explains this benefit, but they are also a rich source of arginine. By increasing nitric oxide levels, arginine may help to improve blood flow, reduce blood clot formation, and improve blood fluidity (the blood becomes thinner and therefore flows through blood vessels more easily).

Walnuts appear to be especially beneficial because they are also a rich source of both antioxidants and alpha-linolenic acid. One study randomly assigned men and women with high cholesterol to either a cholesterol-lowering Mediterranean diet or a diet of similar energy and fat content in which walnuts replaced approximately 32% of the energy from monounsaturated fat (olive oil). Participants followed each diet for four weeks. Compared with the Mediterranean diet, the walnut diet improved endothelial cell function (it increased endothelium-dependent vasodilation and reduced levels of vascular cell adhesion molecule-1). The walnut diet also significantly reduced total cholesterol (a decrease of 4.4%) and LDL (a decrease of 6.4%).[14]

VEGETABLES, FRUIT, AND RED WINE

An important contributor to the benefits noted with the Mediterranean diet is the focus on carotenoid- and flavonoid-rich fruit, vegetables, and beverages (e.g., red wine). Numerous population studies have repeatedly demonstrated that a higher intake of dietary antioxidants significantly reduces the risk of heart disease and stroke. Higher blood levels of antioxidant nutrients from dietary and supplemental sources are also associated with lower levels of hsCRP.[15,16] The importance of antioxidant intake in the prevention and treatment of CAD is discussed further below.

Two valuable sources of antioxidants in the Mediterranean diet are tomato products and red wine. Tomatoes are a rich source of the carotene lycopene. In large clinical studies evaluating the relationship between carotene status and heart attack, lycopene, but not beta carotene, was shown to be protective. Lycopene exerts greater antioxidant activity than beta carotene in general but specifically against LDL oxidation.[17]

The cardiovascular protection offered by red wine is popularly referred to as the "French paradox." Because the French consume more saturated fat

FLAXSEED OIL

In addition to taking a high-quality fish oil, I think it's also a good idea to take a tablespoon of flaxseed oil daily. Flaxseed oil is unique because it contains monounsaturated fatty acid as well as appreciable amounts of the essential fatty acids alpha-linolenic (the essential omega-3 fatty acid) and linoleic acid (the essential omega-6 fatty acid). The best way to take flaxseed oil is by adding it to foods. Don't cook with flaxseed oil – use olive or canola oil. Because flaxseed oil is easily damaged by heat and light, you must add it to foods after cooking.

Taking flaxseed oil by the tablespoon is not very palatable. I recommend trying to incorporate it into your food as much as possible. You can use it as a salad dressing, dip bread into it, add it to hot or cold cereal, or spray it over popcorn. Here is a sample salad dressing featuring flaxseed oil:

FLAXSEED OIL BASIC SALAD DRESSING
This recipe is quick and delicious!

4 tbsp organic flaxseed oil
1½ tbsp lemon juice
1 medium garlic clove, crushed
Pinch of seasoned salt or salt-free seasoning
Fresh ground pepper to taste

Place all ingredients in a bowl and whisk together until smooth and creamy. Jazz up this basic recipe to your personal taste by using your favorite herbs and spices.

than people in the United States and the United Kingdom yet have a lower incidence of heart disease, red wine consumption has been suggested as the reason. Presumably this protection is the result of flavonoids and other polyphenols in red wine that protect against oxidative damage to LDL, as well as helping to reduce the levels of inflammatory mediators.[18] However, moderate alcohol consumption alone has been shown to be protective in some studies by exerting positive effects on the HDL:LDL ratio and CRP as well as levels of fibrinogen, although red wine typically exerts the most significant effects.[19] Importantly, the effects of alcohol on CVD risk, morbidity, and total mortality are counterbalanced by alcohol's addictive and psychological effects and excessive consumption resulting in depletion of glutathione and increased risk of colon cancer.

The major benefit of red wine consumption in protecting against CVD may ultimately be the effect that the polyphenols have on improving the function of the cells that line the blood vessels (endothelial cells).[20] The consumption of green tea and dark chocolate, like that of red wine, has also been shown in population studies to be associated with a reduced risk for CVD. As with red wine, much of the benefit of green tea and chocolate consumption may be the result of several different mechanisms, including improving endothelial cell function.[21]

Other foods and beverages rich in antioxidants have shown benefit in fighting atherosclerosis (hardening of the arteries). Pomegranate (*Punica granatum*) juice appears to be particularly useful. It is remarkably rich in antioxidants, such as soluble polyphenols, tannins, and anthocyanins. Research has indicated that components of pomegranate juice can retard atherosclerosis, reduce plaque formation, and improve arterial health at an intake of 8 oz daily.[22–24]

EAT A "RAINBOW" DIET

One of the best ways to ensure an adequate intake of dietary antioxidants is to focus on eating a "rainbow" assortment of fruit and vegetables regularly. "Rainbow" simply means that selecting colorful foods – red, orange, yellow,

green, blue, and purple – provides the body with the full spectrum of pigments with powerful antioxidant effects as well as the nutrients it needs for
optimal function and protection against disease (Table 2.1).

TAKE GRAPE SEED
OR PINE BARK EXTRACT

One of the most beneficial groups of plant flavonoids are the proanthocyanidins,
also referred to as procyanidins or procyanidolic oligomers (PCOs). Although
PCOs exist in many plants as well as in red wine, commercially available sources
of PCOs include extracts from grape seeds and the bark of the maritime (Landes)
pine. These extracts offer protection to the heart and vascular system via several
different mechanisms, including their antioxidant activity and effects on the
endothelial cells that line blood vessels. PCOs have shown significant benefits in
clinical studies, as antioxidant therapy and for the following health conditions:

* Asthma
* Atherosclerosis, high blood pressure, metabolic syndrome, and
  type 2 diabetes
* Attention deficit disorder
* Male infertility
* Osteoarthritis
* Periodontal disease
* Varicose veins, venous insufficiency, and capillary fragility
* Visual dysfunction, retinopathy, and macular degeneration

Studies show that supplementation with PCOs for six weeks at dosages of
150–300 mg considerably improves the total antioxidant capacity in the blood.
Because of this effect (and others) it simply makes a lot of sense to supplement
at this level on a daily basis with either grape seed extract or pine bark extract.

Table 2.1 The Rainbow Assortment

Red	Dark Green	Yellow and Light Green	Orange	Blue and Purple
Apples (red)	Artichokes	Apples (green or yellow)	Apricots	Beets
Bell peppers (red)	Asparagus	Avocados	Bell peppers (orange)	Blackberries
Cherries	Bell peppers (green)	Bananas	Butternut squash	Blueberries
Cranberries	Broccoli	Bell peppers (yellow)	Cantaloupe	Cabbage (purple)
Grapefruit	Brussels sprouts	Bok choy	Carrots	Cherries
Grapes (red)	Chard	Cabbage	Mangoes	Currants
Plums (red)	Collard greens	Cauliflower	Oranges	Eggplant
Radishes	Cucumbers	Celery	Papaya	Grapes (purple)
Raspberries	Green beans	Fennel	Pumpkin	Onions (red)
Strawberries	Grapes (green)	Kiwi fruit	Sweet potatoes	Pears (red)
Tomatoes	Honeydew melon	Lemons	Yams	Plums (purple)
Watermelon	Kale	Lettuce (light green types)		
	Leeks	Limes		
	Lettuce (dark green types)	Onions		
	Mustard greens	Pears (green or yellow)		
	Peas	Pineapple		
	Spinach	Squash (yellow)		
	Turnip greens	Zucchini (yellow)		

KEEP SALT INTAKE LOW, POTASSIUM INTAKE HIGH

Electrolytes – potassium, sodium, chloride, and magnesium – are mineral salts that can conduct electricity when dissolved in water. For optimal health, it is important to consume these nutrients in the proper balance. Too much sodium in the diet from salt (sodium chloride) can disrupt this balance. Many people know that a high-sodium, low-potassium diet can cause high

EASY TIPS TO REACH YOUR GOAL OF FIVE SERVINGS OF FRUIT AND VEGETABLES PER DAY

- Buy many kinds of fruit and vegetables when you shop so you have plenty of choices.

- Stock up on frozen vegetables for easy cooking so that you always have a vegetable dish with every dinner.

- Use the fruit and vegetables that go bad quickly (peaches, asparagus) first. Save hardier varieties (apples, acorn squash) or frozen goods for later in the week.

- Keep fruit and vegetables where you can see them. The more often you see them, the more likely you are to eat them.

- Keep a bowl of cut-up vegetables on the top shelf of the refrigerator.

- Make a big tossed salad with several kinds of greens, cherry tomatoes, cut up carrots, red pepper, broccoli, scallions and sprouts. Refrigerate in a large glass bowl with an air-tight lid so a delicious mixed salad will be ready to enjoy for several days.

- Keep a fruit bowl on your kitchen counter, table, or desk at work.

- Treat yourself to a fruit sundae. Top a bowl full of your favorite cut-up fruits with vanilla yogurt, shredded coconut, and a handful of nuts.

- Pack a piece of fruit or some cut-up vegetables in your briefcase or backpack; carry moist towelettes for easy cleanup.

- Add fruit and vegetables to lunch by having them in soup, salad, or cut-up raw.

- Use thinly sliced pears or apples in your next omelet.

- At dinner, serve steamed or microwaved vegetables.

- Increase portions when you serve vegetables. One easy way of doing so is adding fresh greens such as Swiss chard, collards, or beet greens to stir fries.

- Choose fresh fruit for dessert. For a special dessert, try a fruit parfait with low-fat yogurt or sherbet topped with lots of berries.

- Add extra varieties of vegetables when you prepare soups, sauces, and casseroles (for example, add grated carrots and zucchini to spaghetti sauce).

- Take advantage of salad bars, which offer ready-to-eat raw vegetables and fruit and prepared salads made with fruit and vegetables.

- Use vegetable-based sauces, such as marinara, and juices such as low-sodium vegetable cocktail or tomato juice.

- Freeze lots of blueberries. They make a great summer replacement for ice cream, ice pops, and other sugary foods.

blood pressure and that the opposite can lower blood pressure,[25,26] but not as many are aware that the former diet also raises the risk of cancer.[27]

In the United States, only 5% of sodium intake comes from the natural ingredients in food. Prepared foods contribute 45% of our sodium intake, 45% is added during cooking, and another 5% is added as a condiment. You can reduce your salt intake by following these tips:

- Take the salt shaker off the table.

- Omit added salt from recipes and food preparation.

- If you absolutely must have the taste of salt, try salt substitutes such as AlsoSalt, NoSalt, and Nu-Salt. These products are made with potassium chloride and taste very similar to sodium chloride.

- Learn to enjoy the flavors of unsalted foods.

- Try flavoring foods with herbs, spices, and lemon juice.

- Read food labels carefully to determine the amounts of sodium. Learn to recognize ingredients that contain sodium. Salt, soy sauce, salt brine, and any ingredient with "sodium" as part of its name, such as monosodium glutamate or baking soda (sodium bicarbonate), contain sodium.

- When reading labels and menus, look for words that signal high sodium content, such as smoked, barbecued, pickled, broth, soy sauce, teriyaki, Creole sauce, marinated, cocktail sauce, tomato base, Parmesan, and mustard sauce.

- Do not eat canned vegetables or soups, which are often extremely high in sodium.

- Choose low-salt (reduced-sodium) products when available.

Most Americans have a potassium to sodium (K:Na) ratio of less than 1:2. In other words, they ingest twice as much sodium as potassium. But experts believe that the optimal dietary potassium to sodium ratio is greater than 5:1—10 times higher than the average intake. However, even this may not be optimal. A natural diet rich in fruit and vegetables can easily produce much higher K:Na ratios, because most fruit and vegetables have a K:Na ratio of at least 50:1. The average K:Na ratios for several common fresh fruits and vegetables are as follows:

- Bananas: 440:1
- Potatoes: 110:1
- Carrots: 75:1
- Oranges: 260:1
- Apples: 90:1

MAGNESIUM

Magnesium is absolutely essential to the proper functioning of the entire cardiovascular system. Its critical role in preventing heart disease and strokes is now widely accepted. In addition, there is a substantial body of knowledge demonstrating that supplementation with magnesium, potassium, or both is effective in treating a wide range of CVDs, including angina, arrhythmia, congestive heart failure, and high blood pressure. In many of these applications, supplementation with magnesium or potassium, or both, has been used for more than 50 years.

The average intake of magnesium by healthy adults in the United States is 143–266 mg/day. This level is well below even the recommended daily allowance (RDA) of 350 mg for men and 300 mg for women. Food choices are the main reason. Because magnesium occurs abundantly in whole foods, most nutritionists and dietitians assume that most Americans get enough magnesium in their diets. But most Americans are not eating whole, natural foods. They are consuming large quantities of processed foods. Because food processing refines out a large portion of magnesium, most Americans are not getting the RDA for magnesium.

The best dietary sources of magnesium are tofu, legumes, seeds, nuts, whole grains, and green leafy vegetables. Fish, meat, milk, and most commonly eaten fruit are quite low in magnesium. Most Americans consume a low-magnesium diet because their diet is high in low-magnesium foods such as processed foods, meat, and dairy products.

People dying of heart attacks have been shown to have lower heart magnesium levels than people of the same age dying of other causes.[28] Low magnesium levels contribute to atherosclerosis and CVD via many mechanisms, including causing dysfunction of the endothelial cells, resulting in inflammation.[29]

ANTIOXIDANT NUTRIENTS

Although diets rich in antioxidant nutrients have consistently shown tremendous protection against CVD, clinical trials using antioxidant vitamins and minerals have produced inconsistent results.[30,31] This failure may be due to several factors, most importantly the fact that the human antioxidant system is a complex arrangement of interacting components. It is unlikely that any single antioxidant would be proven to be effective, especially in the absence of a supporting cast. Most antioxidants require some sort of "partner" antioxidant, allowing them to work more efficiently. The most salient example of this is the partnership between the two primary antioxidants in the human body – vitamins C and E. Vitamin C is an "aqueous (water) phase" antioxidant, while vitamin E is a "lipid (fat) phase" antioxidant. Although some studies have shown that supplementation with these nutrients reduces atherosclerotic lesions, more protection is likely required to ensure optimal effect.[32]

In addition to vitamin C, vitamin E also requires selenium and coenzyme Q_{10} to work efficiently (discussed in more detail later). Further adding to the shortcomings of many studies on antioxidant nutrients is the lack of consideration of the importance of phytochemicals and plant-derived antioxidants that, in addition to being beneficial on their own, are well known to enhance the activities of vitamin and mineral antioxidants.

VITAMIN E AND SELENIUM

Clinical studies have shown inconsistent effects for vitamin E.[33] This could be a result of a lack of selenium or other cofactor for proper vitamin E action. Low levels of selenium are associated with increased risk for CVD.[34] While vitamin E does play a role in protecting against oxidation of LDL, what is probably of greatest importance is to use vitamin E within the context of a comprehensive dietary and supplementation strategy to boost antioxidant status, such as the strategy recommended in this chapter. In this context, vitamin E supplementation definitely plays a role in protecting against heart disease and strokes by its ability to do the following:

- Reduce LDL peroxidation and increase plasma LDL breakdown

- Inhibit excessive platelet aggregation

- Increase HDL levels

- Reduce CRP levels

- Improve endothelial cell function

- Improve insulin sensitivity

VITAMIN C

A high dietary intake of vitamin C has been shown to significantly reduce the risk of death from heart attacks and strokes in numerous population studies. One of the most detailed studies providing insight analyzed the vitamin C intake of 11,348 adults over five years and divided them into three groups:

1. Less than 50 mg daily dietary vitamin C intake.

2. Greater than 50 mg daily dietary vitamin C intake with no vitamin C supplementation.

3. Greater than 50 mg daily dietary vitamin C intake plus vitamin C supplementation (estimated to be 300 mg or more).[35]

Analysis showed that the average death rate was up to 48% lower in the high vitamin C intake group than in the low-intake group for CVD and overall mortality. These differences correspond to an increase in longevity of 5–7 years for men and 1–3 years for women.

Vitamin C works as an antioxidant in aqueous (water-based) environments in the body, both outside and inside human cells. Vitamin C has also been shown to be extremely effective in preventing LDL from being oxidized, even in smokers.[36] Vitamin C and E supplementation of 500 mg and 272 IU daily, respectively, for six years has been shown to reduce the progression of carotid atherosclerosis by 53% in men and 14% in women.[32]

Dozens of observational and clinical studies have shown that vitamin C levels correspond to total cholesterol and HDL. One of the best-designed studies showed that the higher the vitamin C content of the blood, the lower the total cholesterol and triglycerides and the higher the HDL.[37] The benefits for HDL were particularly impressive. For each 0.5 mg/dl increase in vitamin C content of the blood, there was an increase in HDL of 14.9 mg/dl in women and 2.1 mg/dl in men. This study is significant in that it demonstrated that the association of vitamin C and HDL levels persists even in well-nourished individuals with normal serum levels of vitamin C who supplement their diets with additional vitamin C.

IN SUMMARY, VITAMIN C LOWERS THE RISK OF CVD BY DOING THE FOLLOWING:

- Acting as an antioxidant
- Strengthening the collagen structures of the arteries
- Lowering total cholesterol, lipoprotein(a), and blood pressure
- Raising HDL levels
- Inhibiting platelet aggregation
- Promoting fibrinolysis
- Reducing markers of inflammation
- Regenerating vitamin E

TAKE A HIGH-QUALITY MULTIVITAMIN AND MINERAL FORMULA

The best way to get the necessary antioxidant nutrients, such as vitamin C and E, selenium, and beta carotene, as well as other critical nutrients such as magnesium, is by taking a high-quality multivitamin and mineral supplement. Think of it as a nutritional "insurance formula." As noted in the previous chapter, taking a multivitamin and mineral supplement reduces hsCRP levels and may help prevent heart disease. The following recommendations provide an optimum intake range to guide you in selecting a high-quality multi. (Note that vitamins and minerals are measured in different units: IU = International Units, mg = milligrams, and mcg = micrograms.)

Vitamin	Daily Dose for Adults
Vitamin A (retinol)[a]	2500–5000 IU
Vitamin A (from beta carotene)	5000–25,000 IU
Vitamin B$_1$ (thiamin)	10–100 mg
Vitamin B$_2$ (riboflavin)	10–50 mg
Vitamin B$_3$ (niacin)	10–100 mg
Vitamin B$_5$ (pantothenic acid)	25–100 mg
Vitamin B$_6$ (pyridoxine)	25–100 mg
Vitamin B$_{12}$ (methyl cobalamin)	400 mcg
Vitamin C (ascorbic acid)[b]	250–1000 mg
Vitamin D[c]	1000–2000 IU
Vitamin E (mixed tocopherols)[d]	100–200 IU
Vitamin K$_1$ or K$_2$	60–300 mcg
Biotin	100–300 mcg
Choline	10–100 mg
Folic acid	400 mcg
Inositol	10–100 mg
Niacinamide	10–30 mg
Minerals	**Range for Adults**
Boron	1–6 mg
Calcium[e]	250–1000 mg
Chromium[f]	200–400 mcg
Copper	1–2 mg
Iodine	50–150 mcg
Iron[g]	15–30 mg
Magnesium	250–500 mg
Manganese	3–5 mg
Molybdenum	10–25 mcg
Potassium	N/A[h]
Selenium	100–200 mcg
Silica	1–25 mg
Vanadium	50–100 mcg
Zinc	15–30 mg

NOTES

a Women of childbearing age who may become pregnant should not take more than 2500 IU retinol daily because of the possible risk of birth defects.

b It may be easier to take vitamin C separately.

c Elderly people in nursing homes living in northern latitudes should supplement at the high end of the range.

d It may be more cost effective to take vitamin E separately rather than as a component of a multivitamin.

e Women who have or who are at risk of osteoporosis may need to take a separate calcium supplement to achieve the recommended level of 1000 mg daily.

f For diabetes and weight loss, doses of 600 mcg of chromium can be used.

g Most men, as well as most women who have gone through menopause, rarely need supplemental iron.

h The Food and Drug Administration restricts the amount of potassium in supplements to no more than 99 mg. Potassium needs are best met through diet and the use of potassium salts used as a salt substitute.

Read labels carefully to find multivitamin/mineral formulas that contain doses in these ranges. Be aware that you will not find a formula that provides all of these nutrients at these levels in a single pill – it would simply be too big. Most people will need to take at least 3–6 tablets per day to meet these levels. While many "one-a-day" supplements provide good levels of vitamins, they tend to be insufficient in the amount of some of the minerals they provide. Your body needs the minerals as much as the vitamins – the two work hand-in-hand.

WHEN TO TAKE YOUR SUPPLEMENTS

- Multivitamin and mineral supplements are best taken with meals. Whether you take them at the beginning or end of a meal is up to you. If you are taking more than a couple of pills, you may find that taking them at the beginning of a meal is more comfortable. Taking a handful of pills on a full stomach may cause a little stomach upset.

- Flavonoid-rich herbal extracts can be taken with meals or anytime desired.

- Green drinks make great between-meal snacks (especially if you are trying to lose a little weight, as they can quell an overactive appetite).

- Fish oil supplements are best taken at or near the beginning of a meal to avoid any fishy aftertaste — some people burp up a little of the oil if they take it at the end of the meal on a full stomach.

- Vitamin D3 is best taken with meals.

VITAMIN D

Another useful supplement consideration to protect against heart disease is vitamin D. A huge and growing amount of research has now shown that in the U.S. vitamin D deficiency is very common (at least 50% of the general population and 80% of infants) and that it plays a major role in the development in many of the chronic degenerative diseases, including heart disease.[38,39]

Data from a detailed study involving over 8,000 people indicates that individuals with vitamin D (25-OH) levels below 30 ng/ml had a much higher risk for CVD.[38] Another study of more than 3,000 men and women found that those with low vitamin D blood levels had a more than twofold increase in CVD mortality.[39]

The ideal method for determining vitamin D status is a readily available blood test for 25-hydroxyvitamin D_3, or 25(OH)D_3. While some people can achieve an optimal level with just 600 IU per day (or 20 minutes of daily sunlight exposure), others have a genetic requirement for as much 10,000 IU per day. The only way to determine where you fall is by testing. Many doctors are now routinely checking the vitamin D status of their patients. You can also order a test from vitaminDcouncil.org. To take the test, collect a small blood sample by skin prick and send it to the lab. For optimum health, 25(OH)D3 blood levels should be around 50–80 ng/ml (125–200 nmol/l).

If you prefer to just "wing it," take a daily dosage of 1000–2000 IU of vitamin D.

RISK FACTORS FOR VITAMIN D DEFICIENCY

- **INSUFFICIENT EXPOSURE TO SUNLIGHT:** Working and playing indoors, covering up with clothes or sunscreen when outside, and residing at a high latitude reduce exposure to the sun.

- **AGING:** Seniors are at greater risk because of lack of mobility and skin that is less responsive to ultraviolet light.

- **DARKER SKIN:** People of African descent are at greatest risk of vitamin D deficiency owing to higher skin melanin content.

- **BREASTFEEDING:** Breastfeeding will result in vitamin D deficiency in the baby if the mother fails to ensure that her own levels are high enough to provide for her baby's needs.

- **OBESITY:** Fat-soluble vitamin D gets trapped in fat tissue, preventing its utilization by the body.

FINAL COMMENTS

Here is a summary of the key recommendations given in this chapter.

DIETARY RECOMMENDATIONS

- Follow the guidelines of the traditional Mediterranean diet. Specifically, it is important to do the following:

- Consume less saturated fat and cholesterol by reducing or eliminating the amount of animal products you eat.

- Increase your consumption of fiber-rich and antioxidant-rich plant foods (fruit, vegetables, grains, legumes, and raw nuts and seeds).

- Increase your consumption of monounsaturated fats (e.g., nuts, seeds, and olive oil) and omega-3 fatty acids.

- Follow a low-glycemic-load diet.

- Eat a rainbow assortment of fruit and vegetables to ensure a high intake of plant pigments.

- Take one tablespoon of flaxseed oil daily.

- Increase your intake of potassium-rich foods while decreasing your intake of sodium.

NUTRITIONAL SUPPLEMENTS

- Take fish oil: a minimum of 1000 mg EPA+DHA daily.

- Take a high-potency multivitamin and mineral formula according to the guidelines given above. Key individual nutrients include:

  - Vitamin C: 250–500 mg 1–3 times daily

  - Vitamin E (mixed tocopherols): 100–200 IU daily

  - Vitamin D: 1000–2000 IU daily

  - Vitamin B_6: 25–50 mg daily

  - Folic acid: 800 mcg daily

  - Vitamin B_{12}: 800 mcg daily

  - Magnesium: 250–400 mg daily

  - Choose one of the following:

  - Grape seed extract (more than 95% procyanidolic oligomers): 150–300 mg daily

  - Pine bark extract (more than 90% procyanidolic oligomers): 150–300 mg daily

CHAPTER 3

THE TRUTH ABOUT STATINS, CHOLESTEROL, AND NATURAL ALTERNATIVES

The evidence overwhelmingly demonstrates that elevated cholesterol and triglyceride levels greatly increase the risk of death due to cardiovascular disease (CVD). Yet while the drug companies would like us all to believe that it's as simple as taking a statin drug to reduce your risk of a heart attack or stroke, it's just not that simple. Cholesterol-lowering statin drugs are sold primarily under the premise that they will save lives by lowering cholesterol levels, but in reality they have not demonstrated an ability to extend life in over 80% of the patient population these drugs are currently prescribed for.

Annual sales of these drugs now exceed $25 billion. They are a huge profit generator for the drug companies. Without a doubt the creation of the statin drug empire is perhaps the greatest accomplishment of the modern drug era. But this is an achievement the drug companies and doctors should be ashamed of.

While high cholesterol is an important risk factor, it is important to note that more than half of people dying from a heart attack or stroke have low to normal cholesterol levels. The drug companies' and government's response to this fact is to lower the suggested target cholesterol levels even further, thereby effectively casting an even wider net for potential customers. Their goal is to turn all of us into patients hooked on statins. It is very interesting that six of the nine expert members of a government panel that drafted the new cholesterol guidelines had either received grants from or were paid consulting or speakers' fees by the companies that make some of the most popular statin drugs.

Before more fully addressing what the data really tells us about the efficacy and safety of statins, let's first take a closer look at cholesterol and its role in CVD.

WHAT IS CHOLESTEROL?

Cholesterol is a waxy, fat-like substance that has many critical functions in the body. It's found in all cells of the body, where it functions as a necessary structural component of cell membranes. Cholesterol is also used by the body to make many hormones, particularly the sex hormones estrogen and testosterone, but also adrenal hormones such as cortisol and aldosterone. The body also uses cholesterol to make vitamin D. Cholesterol is far from a "bad" substance – it's actually very important to our health.

Cholesterol is transported in the blood on carrier molecules known as lipoproteins. The major categories of lipoproteins are very-low-density lipoprotein (VLDL), low-density lipoprotein (LDL), and high-density lipoprotein (HDL). Since VLDL and LDL are responsible for transporting fats (primarily triglycerides and cholesterol) from the liver to body cells, while HDL is responsible for returning fats to the liver, elevations of either VLDL or LDL are associated with an increased risk for developing atherosclerosis (hardening of the arteries), the primary cause of heart attacks and strokes. In contrast, elevations of HDL are associated with a low risk of heart attacks.

RECOMMENDED BLOOD CHOLESTEROL LEVELS

It is currently recommended that the total blood cholesterol level be less than 200 mg/dl and triglyceride levels be lower than 150 mg/dl. In addition, it is recommended that the LDL cholesterol level be less than 130 mg/dl and HDL cholesterol greater than 35 mg/dl.

The total cholesterol to HDL and LDL:HDL ratios are referred to as the cardiac risk factor ratios because they reflect whether cholesterol is being deposited into tissues or broken down and excreted. The total cholesterol to HDL ratio should be no higher than 4.2, and the LDL:HDL ratio should be no higher than 2.5. The risk for heart disease can be reduced dramatically by lowering LDL while simultaneously raising HDL levels: For every 1% drop in the LDL level, the risk for a heart attack drops by 2%. Conversely, for every 1% increase in HDL levels, the risk for a heart attack drops 3–4%.

Although LDL is referred to as "bad cholesterol," there are some forms that are worse than others. For example, oxidized LDL is a persistent pro-inflammatory trigger for the progression of atherosclerosis and plaque rupture. LDL molecules of higher density are associated with greater risk than larger, less dense LDL. Small, dense LDL are more likely to cause atherosclerosis than are larger and less dense LDL, and are markers for CVD risk.[1] The reason is that these smaller particles (LDL3) are more likely to be attached with sugar molecules (glycated) over the larger, more buoyant LDL. This highlights again the importance of avoiding high blood sugar levels and subsequent glycation.[2]

Another marker that deserves mention is lipoprotein (a), or Lp(a), a plasma lipoprotein whose structure and composition closely resemble those of LDL, but with an additional molecule of an adhesive protein called apolipoprotein(a). Elevated plasma levels of Lp(a) are an independent risk factor for coronary heart disease, particularly in patients with elevated LDL levels. In fact, in one analysis a high level of Lp(a) was shown to carry with it a 10 times greater risk for heart disease than an elevated LDL level.[3] That's because LDL on its own lacks the adhesive apolipoprotein(a). As a result, LDL does not easily stick to the walls of the artery. Actually, a high LDL level carries less risk than a normal or even low LDL with high Lp(a). Levels of Lp(a) below 20 mg/dl are associated with a low risk for heart disease, levels of 20–40 mg/dl are associated with a moderate risk, and levels above 40 mg/dl are associated with an extremely high risk for heart disease.

ELEVATIONS OF TRIGLYCERIDES

In the past, the relation between elevations in blood triglycerides (hypertri-glyceridemia) and coronary heart disease (CHD) has been uncertain. However, a large body of accumulating evidence indicates that high triglycerides are an independent risk factor for cardiovascular disease.[4,5] When high triglycerides are combined with elevations in LDL, it's a recipe for an early heart attack. In one analysis, high triglycerides combined with elevated LDL and a high LDL:HDL cholesterol ratio (above 5) increased the CHD event risk approximately sixfold.

Table 3.1 Recommended Cholesterol and Triglyceride Levels

Lipid Type	Level (mg/dl)	Result
Total cholesterol	Less than 200	Desirable
	200–239	Borderline
	240 or more	High risk
LDL cholesterol	Less than 100*	Desirable
	100–130	Borderline
	130–159	Borderline high risk
	160 or more	High risk

Lipid Type	Level (mg/dl)	Result
HDL cholesterol	Less than 35	Low (undesirable)
	35–59	Normal
	60 or more	Desirable
Triglycerides	Less than 150	Desirable
	150–199	Borderline high
	200–499	High
	500 or more	Very high

*For very-high-risk patients (those having signs and symptoms of CVD, a prior cardiovascular event, or with multiple risk factors such as diabetes, continued smoking, and high blood pressure), an LDL of less than 70 mg/dl is often recommended.

INHERITED ELEVATIONS OF CHOLESTEROL AND TRIGLYCERIDES

Elevations of blood cholesterol, triglycerides, or both can be due to genetic factors. These conditions are referred to as familial high cholesterol, familial combined hyperlipidemia (FCH), and familial high triglycerides. Relatively speaking, these disorders are among the most common inherited diseases – they affect about one in every 500 people.

The basic problem in familial high cholesterol is a defect in the receptor protein for LDL in the liver. Under normal situations the LDL receptor is responsible for removing cholesterol from the blood. When a liver cell takes up LDL after it has bound to a receptor, the LDL signals the liver cell to stop making cholesterol. In familial high cholesterol the defect in the LDL receptor results in the liver not receiving the message to stop making cholesterol.

Damage to the LDL receptor occurs with normal aging and in several disease states, diabetes chief among them because of increased glycosylation of the receptor proteins. As a result of LDL receptor damage, cholesterol levels tend to rise with age. In addition, a diet high in saturated fat and cholesterol decreases the number of LDL receptors, thereby reducing the feedback mechanism that tells the liver cell that no more cholesterol is necessary.

Fortunately, lifestyle and dietary changes can increase the function or number of LDL receptors, or both. The most dramatic effects are in people without inherited causes of elevated cholesterol or triglycerides, but even people with familial high cholesterol can benefit.

FCH and familial high triglycerides result in defects similar to familial high cholesterol. In FCH the basic defect appears to be an accelerated production of VLDL in the liver. These individuals may have only a high blood triglyceride level or only a high cholesterol level, or both. In familial high triglycerides there is only an elevation in blood triglyceride levels, and HDL levels tend to be low. The defect in familial high triglycerides is that the VLDL particles made by the liver are larger than normal and carry more triglycerides. Familial high triglycerides is made worse by diabetes, gout, and obesity.

LOWERING CHOLESTEROL

Lowering total cholesterol, as well as LDL and triglycerides, is clearly associated with reducing CVD risk. Most of the benefits noted with lowering LDL are based on a large number of randomized clinical trials involving the use of 3-hydroxy-3 methylglutaryl coenzyme A (HMG-CoA) reductase inhibitors known collectively as statin drugs. Statin drugs owe their origin to red yeast *(Monascus purpureus)* fermented on rice.

This traditional Chinese medicine has been used for its health-promoting effects in China for more than 2,000 years. Red yeast rice is the source of a group of compounds known as monacolins (e.g., lovastatin, also known as monacolin K, one of the key monacolins in red yeast rice extract). The marketing of an extract of red yeast fermented on rice standardized for monacolin content as a dietary supplement in the United States caused controversy in 1997 because it contained a natural source of a prescription drug. The Food and Drug Administration eventually ruled that red yeast rice products could be sold only if they were free of monacolin content.

THE STATIN DRUG EMPIRE

The statin drug empire consists of popular cholesterol-lowering drugs such as Crestor (rosuvastatin), Lipitor (atorvastatin), Zocor (simvastatin), Mevacor (lovastatin), and Pravachol (pravastatin), along with similar drugs that lower cholesterol by inhibiting an enzyme in the liver (HMG-CoA reductase) that manufactures cholesterol. Annual sales of these drugs now exceed $25 billion. Millions of prescriptions are filled yearly with the hope of reducing people's risk of developing heart disease.

But looking at the results of detailed studies, the majority of people on statin drugs are deriving no real benefit from them. In fact, relying on these drugs and not focusing on effectively reducing heart disease risk through diet, lifestyle, and proper nutritional supplementation is costing many people their lives. In addition, while drug companies and many doctors state that statins are so safe and effective they should be added to drinking water, the reality is that they are very expensive medicines, provide very limited benefit, and carry with them considerable risks for side effects. For example, a 2012 study by the Mayo Clinic found that the use of statins in postmenopausal women increased their risk for type 2 diabetes by 74%.[6] Some of the other side effects noted with statins include the following:

- Liver problems and decreased liver function

- Interference with the manufacture of coenzyme Q_{10} (CoQ_{10}), a key substance responsible for energy production within the body

- Rhabdomyolysis, the breaking down of muscle tissue, which can be fatal

- Nerve damage – the chances of nerve damage are 26 times higher in statin users than in the general population

- Impaired mental function with prolonged use

- Possible increased risk of cancer and heart failure with long-term use

- Increased muscle damage caused by exercise and reduced exercise capacity

- Worsening energy levels and fatigue after exertion in about 20% of cases

The medical consensus, based on numerous long-term studies, has now shown quite convincingly that in people with a history of a heart attack, stroke, or current signs and symptoms of existing CVD, statins do produce some benefits in reducing deaths due to a heart attack, but the overall effect on life expectancy remains somewhat controversial. In other words, the drugs reduce deaths due to heart attacks, but overall life expectancy is no different than in the placebo group. For example, in the large Heart Protection Study, men with CVD taking a statin for five years only reduced their chances of death from 15% to 13%.[7] The reduced rate of heart attacks and strokes may be offset by an increase in other causes of death (e.g., possibly cancer).

The larger issue is whether statins produce any benefit in people without evidence of CVD. About 75% of the prescriptions for statins are written for people with no clinical evidence of CVD. So, while there is some evidence, though not all that impressive, in the prevention of a second heart attack (secondary prevention), the benefit of statins in preventing a first heart attack or stroke (primary prevention) has not been proven to any sufficient standard. So, the writing of prescriptions for statins for the primary prevention of death due to CVD is not consistent with scientific studies. If your doctor is pushing a statin on you even though you have no evidence of CVD, he or she is simply not practicing evidence-based medicine.

Large evaluations of studies in people without a history of heart attack or stroke who took statin drugs and lowered their cholesterol have shown they did not live any longer than the people in the placebo group.[8–11] For example, the largest and most thorough review of statins analyzed 11 clinical trials involving 65,229 participants and was published in the *Archives of Internal Medicine* in June 2010.[11] The analysis provides the most reliable evidence available on the impact of statin therapy on all-cause mortality among high-risk individuals without prior CVD. The results showed that the use of statin therapy did not result in reduction in all-cause mortality in these high-risk patients.

These results are consistent with other quality reviews and call into question the widespread use of statins not only in high-risk patients without CVD, but also in patients with the only risk present being elevated LDL. This issue will be further discussed below.

While there is the occasional positive study with a statin drug showing some benefit in reducing mortality (of course, funded by the drug company), the effect noted pales in comparison with the effect of dietary and lifestyle interventions. For example, one study appearing in *The New England Journal of Medicine* followed the activity level and health of retired men in Honolulu between the ages of 61 and 81.[12] These men were followed for over 10 years and divided into two groups; one group walked less than one mile per day

IS A SIESTA MORE EFFECTIVE THAN A STATIN DRUG?

Taking an afternoon nap (a siesta) is common in populations with low rates of heart attack (coronary) deaths. To study the benefit of a siesta on heart health, researchers carefully selected subjects to prevent confounding variables such as physical activity and diet from interfering with a statistical analysis. The analysis was conducted on results from the Greek European Prospective Investigation into Cancer and Nutrition (EPIC) study involving 23,681 individuals who at enrollment had no history of coronary heart disease, stroke, or cancer and had complete information on frequency and duration of midday napping.[13]

These people were followed for an average of nearly 6.5 years. The results were astounding. People who took a siesta of any frequency or duration had a 34% reduced rate of having a heart attack. Further analysis showed that occasionally napping produced a 12% lower coronary mortality rate, whereas those who regularly napped had a 37% lower coronary mortality. These results are far superior to the results demonstrated with statin drugs in the primary prevention of CVD and raise the question, "Is taking a nap more effective in preventing a heart attack than taking a statin?"

The answer appears to be yes.

while the other group walked more than two miles per day. The group that walked more than two miles per day had almost 50% fewer deaths during that period than those who walked less than one mile per day. Interesting – a drug-free plan that costs nothing offers better benefits on mortality than the high-priced cholesterol-lowering drugs.

A CLOSER LOOK AT HOW STATINS WORK

Statins work by blocking an enzyme (HMG-CoA reductase) that produces a compound (mevalonate) that is the direct precursor to cholesterol (see Figure 3.1). The problem is that statins not only inhibit the production of cholesterol but of a whole host of other substances that have important bodily biochemical functions. Figure 3.1 illustrates the cholesterol pathway and its intermediary products as well as end products that include not only cholesterol but also CoQ_{10} and dolichols.

CoQ_{10} is a critical component in the manufacture of ATP – the energy currency of our cells. Basically, CoQ_{10}'s role in our cells is similar to the role of a spark plug in a car engine. Just as the car cannot function without that initial spark, the cell cannot function without CoQ_{10}. Although the body makes some of its own CoQ_{10}, considerable research shows significant benefits with supplementation. Also, people with any sort of heart disease, including high cholesterol levels and high blood pressure, and those taking cholesterol-lowering drugs are known to have low CoQ_{10} levels.

Since statin drugs reduce the production of CoQ_{10}, taking them would obviously produce some serious consequences, since organs like the heart, liver, muscles, and brain require large amounts of CoQ_{10} to function properly. The research seems to support this observation since the serious side effects of statin drugs appear to be related to lowering CoQ_{10} levels.[14] In addition, deaths attributed to heart failure have nearly doubled since 1989 – an interesting fact since statins first hit the market in a big way in 1988. If you are taking a statin drug, you definitely need to supplement with CoQ_{10} at a dosage of 100–200 mg daily. Choose products in soft gel capsules with rice bran oil for maximum absorption.

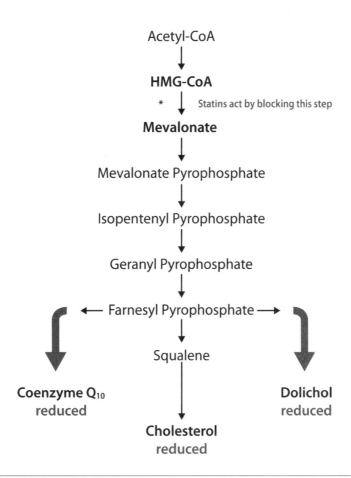

Figure 3.1 Cholesterol manufacture in the liver showing the end products affected by statin drugs.

Another less talked about component of the cholesterol pathway, production of which is also inhibited by statin drugs, is dolichols. Like CoQ_{10}, dolichols are very important in human biology. One of their key functions is to help direct proteins to their targeted cells. In other words, when your liver or other tissue makes certain proteins, those proteins need to be delivered to specific destinations; dolichols make that possible. Since statin drugs can reduce the amounts of dolichols in the circulation, they may be producing significant chaos in our body processes. A good analogy would be having a very large city with no street signs or addresses; mail would never be delivered and outsiders could never find their destinations.

AN HONEST APPRAISAL OF THE BENEFITS OF STATINS IN PRIMARY PREVENTION

There is no question that individuals with clinical evidence of CVD, i.e., signs and symptoms such as angina, shortness of breath, or peripheral artery disease are present, need to be aggressive with lowering of cholesterol and triglycerides, but this does not necessarily mean with a statin. The combination of dietary, lifestyle, and supplement recommendations given in this chapter can easily achieve targets. In the rare cases in which after three months these targets are not met, then a statin may be appropriate in these extremely high risk individuals.

In individuals with moderate risk due to diabetes, high blood pressure, or extremely high cholesterol (LDL higher than 150 mg/dl), again it is important to achieve targets, but nondrug therapies should be attempted for at least three months before opting for a statin. Statins have not been shown to reduce all-cause mortality in this group (see below).

The consensus of expert opinion is that in individuals at low risk or having the only major risk factor of high LDL, statins are not likely to produce any benefit. In fact, doctors have been cautioned against writing prescriptions for statins for these patients, yet the reality is that this group represents a very large percentage of statin users. Your doctor may tell you that a statin will cut your risk for a heart attack or stroke in half. If they do, they are listening too much to the drug company sales rep or propaganda and not thinking for themselves.

The bottom line is that in low-risk patients statins produce no meaningful benefit and carry with them significant risks. It's just not very good medicine and not very cost effective to prescribe statins to this group. Furthermore, I think better results would be produced in actually reducing mortality and extending life by following the guidelines given in Chapter 2, along with those in this chapter, for lowering cholesterol and triglycerides.

The drug companies and most doctors want us to believe that since statins lower cholesterol, they most assuredly reduce the risk of heart attacks and strokes in people without CVD. But the truth is that while there is no question that lower levels of cholesterol equate to a reduced number of deaths due to CVD based on population studies, lowering cholesterol levels *with statins* has not been proven to produce the same risk reduction and increase life expectancy in people *without* CVD, despite a considerable effort by the drug companies. Again, careful review of the major statin drug studies in people without clinical evidence of CVD shows that there are no significant differences in mortality between people who took cholesterol-lowering agents and those who took a placebo. Pooled data from all randomized trials that compared statins with placebo in primary prevention of CVD mortality showed that total mortality was not reduced by statins. For example:

- Data from 11 clinical trials involving 65,229 participants considered high-risk individuals, but without prior heart attack or stroke, showed use of statin therapy did not result in reduction in all-cause mortality.[11]

- Statins did not reduce total heart attacks or strokes in 10,990 women in the primary prevention trials.[15]

- In 3,239 men and women older than 69 years, statins did not reduce total heart attacks or strokes.[16] Use of statins as a primary preventer in this age group is not supported by research.

- In 10,355 patients with high blood pressure who were randomized to receive a placebo or drug therapy using a statin (40 mg/day of pravastatin), there was no significant difference in the rate of death, heart disease, or heart attack.[17]

- In a study involving 47,294 patients without CVD, researchers gave participants either 40 mg of simvastatin or a placebo. There was no correlation between treatment and amount of LDL lowering and death rate.[18]

- Statins may significantly increase the risk of diabetes in postmenopausal women.

The consensus among most medical experts not aligned with or supported by the drug companies is that statins should not be prescribed for the primary prevention of CVD mortality in anyone without prior heart attack or stroke or current clinical signs and symptoms of CVD. Obviously, relying on statin drugs, in lieu of important dietary, lifestyle, and nutritional supplement approaches, just does not make very much sense.

WHY STATINS FAIL

CVD is a multifactorial disease. Trying to simplify it by addressing only one risk factor is doomed to failure. Simply stated, there are significantly more important things to consider than the level of LDL. The whole premise on reducing LDL levels with statins is the faulty belief that it will reduce the buildup of arterial plaque, but researchers at Beth Israel Medical Center in New York City demonstrated the real reason statins do not work.[19]

They examined coronary plaque buildup in patients who took statins at a dosage of either more than 80 mg/day or less than 80 mg/day. At the beginning of the study all patients had their coronary arterial plaques measured using electron beam tomography. At the end of the 12-month study, cholesterol levels and coronary plaques were again measured. Although both groups were successful in lowering their cholesterol, this did not produce any effect in the progression of the plaque buildup. In other words, the buildup of plaque (which is why doctors try to lower cholesterol) didn't appear to be related to blood cholesterol levels.

Again, there are other factors involved in the process of atherosclerosis that are significantly more important than lowering cholesterol, but are largely ignored because they do not involve drug therapy.

DIET VS. STATINS

Dietary measures alone are often extremely effective in lowering cholesterol levels. For example, one interesting study compared the "portfolio diet," comprising plant-based cholesterol-lowering foods, to lovastatin.[20] The participants were randomly assigned to undergo one of three interventions on an outpatient basis for one month: a diet low in saturated fat, based on milled whole-wheat cereals and low-fat dairy foods (the control diet); the same diet plus 20 mg/day lovastatin (the lovastatin diet); or a diet high in plant sterols (1 g/1000 kcal), soy protein (21.4 g/1000 kcal), viscous fibers (9.8 g/1000 kcal), and almonds (14 g/1000 kcal) (the portfolio diet).

The three groups had average decreases in LDL as follows: control diet, 8%; statin diet, 30.9%; and portfolio diet, 28.6%. Respective reductions in C-reactive protein (CRP) were 10%, 33.3%, and 28.2%.

This and subsequent studies show that diversifying cholesterol-lowering components in the same dietary portfolio increased the effectiveness of diet as a treatment for high cholesterol and produced results comparable to those of a statin drug, with lipid-lowering effects similar to statins in terms of both LDL and LDL size, but without the side effects.[21,22]

The key point is that while individual dietary changes may produce benefit in improving blood lipids, the best clinical approach is to incorporate a broad-spectrum dietary approach that incorporates a wide array of dietary components shown to positively affect lipid levels.

Here is another example: A meta-analysis of 27 randomized controlled trials in which isolated soy protein supplementation was the only intervention demonstrated that soy protein supplementation was associated with a significant dose-dependent reduction in serum total cholesterol, LDL, and triglycerides. But the effect shown was less than the effect noted above, in which the soy protein was used in conjunction with other dietary interventions in the portfolio diet.[23] In addition, the effects of isolated soy protein appear to be considerably less than the effect of increasing soy food consumption in general.

Much of the cholesterol-lowering effect of soy foods may relate more to the isoflavone and soluble fiber content than to the protein. In an earlier meta-analysis based more on soy protein intake from other sources in addition to soy protein isolate, reductions were much more significant for total cholesterol (–23.2 mg/dl), LDL (–21.7 mg/dl), and triglycerides (–13.3 mg/dl), but still relatively modest from a clinical perspective.[24]

While these results do support the recommendation to increase soy protein intake as part of the dietary approach to high cholesterol, given the relatively small effect of soy protein on lipids, it is imperative that other dietary recommendations, such as reducing the dietary intake of saturated fat, trans fatty acids, and cholesterol, as well as increasing intake of monounsaturated fats, soluble fiber, and nuts, also be promoted.

THE UPHILL BATTLE

Despite research showing that statins offer no benefit in reducing mortality in patients without a history of CVD, and despite all the research documenting the benefits of nondrug approaches, it is unlikely that lowering LDL with statin drugs will be supplanted as the primary therapy in lipid management and prevention of CAD anytime in the near future. In 2011, it was estimated that more than one of every six adults – nearly 40 million people – were taking a statin drug to lower LDL.

Therefore the focus for many will be on the support of statin therapy. For example, as described above, it is important that individuals taking statin drugs supplement with CoQ_{10}. Researchers have concluded that inhibition of CoQ_{10} synthesis by statin drugs could explain the most commonly reported side effects, especially fatigue and muscle pain, as well as the more serious side effects, such as rhabdomyolysis.[25,26] CoQ_{10} supplementation in people on statin drugs has also been shown to reduce markers of oxidative damage.

CALCULATE THE IMPACT OF LOWERING CHOLESTEROL WITH A STATIN YOURSELF

If you doubt the research I've cited on the failure of statins to reduce the risk of having a heart attack, I encourage you to use the math predicting the risk of having a heart attack in the next 10 years based on cholesterol levels by visiting The National Cholesterol Education Program calculator at hp2010.nhlbihin.net/atpiii/calculator.asp. Just for this exercise, enter data for a 55-year-old nonsmoking woman with total cholesterol of 240 mg/dl (high enough to make most physicians prescribe a statin), HDL of 50 mg/dl (which is quite low for women), and systolic blood pressure of 110 mm Hg. The results should show that this woman has a 1% chance of having a heart attack over the next decade. Now change her total cholesterol to 190 mg/dl – a huge decline. Her risk is still 1%. A 65-year-old man with those first numbers has an 11% chance of having a heart attack over the next decade; lowering his cholesterol to 190 mg/dl brings that down to 9% – not a big drop.

Now enter your own data to see what your risk is. Now, play around with different levels of cholesterol. Not that big of a difference, is there? Why? Well, it turns out that while cholesterol levels are important, they are not as strongly predictive of CVD as once thought or as important as the drug companies would like us to believe. Remember, roughly half of people who have a heart attack do not have high cholesterol levels.

EFFECT OF DIETARY CHOLESTEROL ON CVD RISK

While the liver is the major source of blood cholesterol, dietary cholesterol can be an important contributor. Diets high in cholesterol are associated with an increased risk for heart disease, cancer, and strokes. However, it may be that the level of saturated fats in these foods is more relevant than their cholesterol content.

This opinion is supported by a statistical analysis of 224 dietary studies carried out over the past 25 years that investigated the relationship between diet and blood cholesterol levels in over 8,000 people.[27] What investigators found was that saturated fat in the diet, not dietary cholesterol, is what influences blood cholesterol levels the most. The data indicates that dietary cholesterol in most people has very little effect on blood cholesterol levels. Nonetheless, it is generally recommended that a healthy person should restrict dietary cholesterol intake to 300 mg per day. Someone with high cholesterol or heart disease should consume no more than 200 mg of cholesterol daily. In addition, it is important to keep the daily saturated fat intake to a bare minimum. Certainly, no more than 10–15 g per day is recommended – ideally less.

Table 3.2 Cholesterol and Fat Content of Selected foods

Food	Serving Size	Total Fat (g)	Saturated Fat (g)	Monounsaturated Fat (g)	Polyunsaturated Fat (g)	Cholesterol (mg)
Beef, lean	3 oz.	7.9	3.0	3.3	0.3	73
Beef liver, braised	3 oz.	4.2	1.6	0.6	0.9	331
Chicken breast, roasted	3 oz.	3.0	0.9	1.1	0.6	72
Chicken leg, roasted	3 oz.	7.2	2.0	2.6	1.7	79
Egg yolk	1 large	5.1	1.6	1.9	0.7	213
Fish, cod	3 oz.	0.7	0.1	0.1	0.3	40
Lobster, boiled	3 oz.	0.5	0.1	0.1	0.1	61
Pork, lean	3 oz.	11.1	3.8	5.0	1.3	79
Shrimp, boiled	3 oz.	0.9	0.2	0.2	0.4	166
Turkey, dark, roasted	3 oz.	6.1	2.1	1.4	1.8	73
Turkey, light, roasted	3 oz.	2.7	0.9	0.5	0.7	59
Cheese, cheddar	1 oz.	9.4	6.0	2.7	0.3	30
Ice cream, regular	½ cup	7.2	4.5	2.1	0.3	30
Milk, low fat 2%	1 cup	4.7	2.9	1.4	0.2	18
Milk, skim	1 cup	0.4	0.3	0.1	neg	4
Milk, whole	1 cup	8.2	5.1	2.4	0.3	33
Butter	1 tbsp	11.5	7.2	3.3	0.4	31

IMPORTANCE OF SOLUBLE DIETARY FIBER IN LOWERING CHOLESTEROL

It is well established that the soluble dietary fiber found in legumes, fruit, and vegetables is effective in lowering cholesterol levels.[28] The greater the degree of viscosity or gel-forming nature, the greater the effect a particular dietary fiber has on lowering cholesterol levels.

PGX® is a new, highly viscous, soluble fiber matrix that is showing greater effect than previously used single-source fibers, leading to more reasonable dosage recommendations (the cholesterol-lowering effect of soluble fiber is clearly dose dependent).[29,30] PGX® will be discussed more fully in Chapter 4 for its ability to improve blood sugar control and insulin sensitivity.

Table 3.3 shows the average doses and reductions noted in clinical trials with soluble fiber products, mainly oat preparations containing either oat bran or oatmeal.[31] The overwhelming majority of these studies demonstrated that individuals with high cholesterol levels experience significant reductions with frequent oatmeal or oat bran consumption. In contrast, individuals with normal or low cholesterol levels see little change. In individuals with high cholesterol levels (above 200 mg/dl), the consumption of the equivalent of 3 g of soluble oat fiber typically lowers total cholesterol by 8–23%. This is highly significant, as with each 1% drop in serum cholesterol level there is a 2% decrease in the risk of developing heart disease. Approximately one bowl of ready-to-eat oat bran cereal or oatmeal contains 3 g of fiber. Although oatmeal's fiber content (7%) is less than that of oat bran (15–26%), it has been determined that the polyunsaturated fatty acids it contains contribute as much to the cholesterol-lowering effects of oats as the fiber content. Although oat bran has a higher fiber content, oatmeal is higher in polyunsaturated fatty acids.

In an effort to lower cholesterol with dietary fiber, try to eat 35 g of fiber daily from fiber-rich foods, a full listing of which is found in Appendix A. Achieving higher fiber intake is not only associated with lower cholesterol levels, but also lower inflammatory mediators, such as CRP.[32]

Table 3.3 Impact of Sources of Fiber on Serum Cholesterol Levels

Fiber Dosage (g per day)	Typical Reduction in Total Cholesterol, %
Oat bran (dry), 50–100	15–20
PGX®, 3–15	15–20
Psyllium, 10–20	10–20
Guar gum, 9–15	10
Vegetable fiber, 27	10
Pectin, 6–10	5

FISH OILS TO LOWER TRIGLYCERIDE LEVELS

The benefits of the longer-chain omega-3 fatty acids eicosapentaenoic acid (EPA) and docosahexaenoic acid (DHA) on cardiovascular health have been demonstrated in more than 300 clinical trials. While supplementation with EPA+DHA has little effect on cholesterol levels, it does lower triglyceride levels significantly and produces myriad additional benefits in protecting against CVD.[33] In general, for prevention of CVD, the dosage recommendation is 1000 mg EPA+DHA per day, but for lowering triglycerides the dosage is 3000–5000 mg EPA+DHA.[34]

Lower dosages of EPA+DHA exert only mild effects on triglyceride levels. For example, intakes of 200–500 mg/day lower triglyceride levels by 3.1–7.2%.[35] In one double-blind study, after eight weeks of supplementation a daily dosage of 3400 mg EPA+DHA lowered triglycerides by 27%, while a lower dosage of 850 mg had no significant effect.[36]

These results clearly indicate that the effective dosage for lowering triglycerides with fish oils is 3000 mg EPA+DHA per day. The degree of reduction in triglycerides with fish oil is on par with other drug therapies. For example, in patients with triglyceride levels above 500 mg/dl, approximately 4000 mg/day of EPA+DHA reduces triglyceride levels by 45%. Fish oils work to lower triglyceride levels via several mechanisms that basically reduce the formation of triglycerides while increasing their breakdown into energy.[37]

NATURAL PRODUCTS TO LOWER CHOLESTEROL LEVELS

In many cases dietary therapy, while important, is not sufficient alone to reduce lipid levels to the desired ranges. Fortunately, several natural compounds can lower cholesterol levels and other significant risk factors for CVD. In fact, when all factors are considered (e.g., cost, safety, effectiveness), the natural alternatives presented here may offer significant advantages to the standard drug therapy, especially when used together rather than as isolated therapies.

NIACIN

Since the 1950s niacin (vitamin B3) has been known to be effective in lowering blood cholesterol levels. In the 1970s the famed Coronary Drug Project demonstrated that niacin was the only cholesterol-lowering agent to actually reduce overall mortality. Niacin typically lowers LDL levels by 16–23% while raising HDL levels by 20–33%. These effects, especially the effect on HDL, compare quite favorably with conventional cholesterol-lowering drugs.[38,39]

It is now known that niacin does much more than lower total cholesterol. Specifically, niacin has been shown to lower LDL, the more harmful Lp(a) lipoprotein, triglyceride, CRP, and fibrinogen levels while simultaneously raising beneficial HDL levels. Despite the fact that niacin has demonstrated better overall results in reducing risk factors for CHD than other cholesterol-lowering agents, physicians are often reluctant to prescribe niacin. The reason is a widespread perception that niacin is difficult to work with because of the bothersome flushing of the skin.

In addition, because niacin is a widely available generic product, no pharmaceutical company stands to generate the huge profits that the other lipid-lowering agents have enjoyed. As a result, niacin does not benefit from intensive research and advertising, like statin drugs do. Despite the advantages of niacin over other lipid-lowering drugs, it accounts for less than 10% of all cholesterol-lowering prescriptions. Niaspan, a prescription niacin product, accounted for 952,000 prescriptions in 2002, translating to sales of $145.7 million – a dramatic 73% increase from 2001 levels. By 2010, sales reached over $927 million and approximately 100,000 prescriptions per week. The increasing sales of niacin reflect a growing physician awareness of the advantages of niacin over statin drugs.

Several studies have compared niacin with standard lipid-lowering drugs, including statins. These studies have shown significant advantages for niacin. In the first published clinical study, niacin was compared with lovastatin directly in 136 patients with LDL levels greater than 160 mg/dl and with either CHD or more than two CHD risk factors, or both; or in patients with LDL levels greater than 190 mg/dl and without CHD or with fewer than two CHD risk factors.[40] The controlled, randomized, open-label, 26-week study was performed at five lipid clinics. Patients were first placed on a four-week diet run-in period, after which eligible patients were randomly assigned to receive treatment with either lovastatin (20 mg/day) or niacin (1500 mg/day). On the basis of the LDL response and patient tolerance, the doses were sequentially increased to 40 and 80 mg/day of lovastatin or 3000 and 4500 mg/day of niacin after 10 and 18 weeks of treatment, respectively. In the two patient groups, 66% of patients treated with lovastatin and 54% of patients treated with niacin underwent full dosage increases. Table 3.4 shows the results.

These results indicate that while lovastatin produced a greater LDL reduction, niacin provided better overall results despite the fact that fewer patients were able to tolerate a full dosage of niacin because of skin flushing. The percentage increase in HDL, a more significant indicator for CHD, was dramatically in favor of niacin (33% vs. 7%). Equally impressive was the percentage decrease in Lp(a) for niacin: Niacin produced a 35% reduction in Lp(a) levels, while lovastatin did not produce any effect. Niacin's effect on Lp(a) in this study confirmed a previous study that showed niacin (4000 mg/day) reduced Lp(a) levels by 38%; a subsequent study showed similar reductions in Lp(a) in patients with diabetes.[41,42]

Table 3.4 Comparison of Niacin to Lovastatin

Lipoprotein	Group	Week 10, %	Week 18, %	Week 26, %
LDL cholesterol (reduction)	Lovastatin	26	28	32
	Niacin	5	16	23
HDL cholesterol (increase)	Lovastatin	6	8	7
	Niacin	20	29	33
Lp(a) lipoprotein (reduction)	Lovastatin	0	0	0
	Niacin	14	30	35

Another comparative study evaluated the lipoprotein responses to niacin, gemfibrozil, and lovastatin in patients with normal total cholesterol levels but low levels of HDL.[43] The first phase of the study compared lipoprotein responses with lovastatin and gemfibrozil in 61 middle-aged men with low HDL. In the second phase, 37 patients agreed to take niacin; 27 patients finished this phase at a dose of 4500 mg/day. In the first phase, gemfibrozil therapy increased HDL levels by 10% and lovastatin by 6%. In the second phase, niacin therapy was shown to raise HDL by 30%.

Another study compared niacin with atorvastatin (Lipitor).[44] The average dosage was 3000 mg for niacin and 80 mg for Lipitor. The patients selected had abnormal LDL particle size in that the molecules were small and dense – these LDL molecules are considerably more likely to cause atherosclerosis than are larger, less dense LDL particles. The patients selected also had low levels (less than 40%) of HDL2 – a type of HDL2 associated with greater protection than HDL alone. Although Lipitor reduced total LDL levels substantially more than niacin, niacin was more effective at increasing LDL particle size and raising HDL and HDL2 than Lipitor (Table 3.5).

Table 3.5 Effect of Atorvastatin (Lipitor) and Niacin on Lipid Profiles

Parameter	Atorvastatin		Niacin		Atorvastatin + Niacin	
	Before	After	Before	After	Before	After
Total LDL (mg/dl)	110	56	111	89	123	55
LDL peak diameter (Å)	251	256	253	263	250	263
Lipoprotein(a) (mg/dl)	45	44	37	23	54	35
HDL (mg/dl)	42	43	38	54	38	54
HDL2 (%)	30	42	29	43	32	37
Triglycerides (mg/dl)	186	100	194	108	235	73

Because taking niacin at higher dosages (e.g., ≥3000 mg) can impair glucose tolerance, many physicians have avoided niacin therapy in diabetics, but newer studies with slightly lower dosages (1000–2000 mg) of niacin have not shown it to adversely affect blood sugar regulation.[45] For example, during a 16-week, double-blind, placebo-controlled trial, 148 type 2 diabetes patients were randomized to placebo or 1000 or 1500 mg/day of niacin. In the niacin-treated groups there was no significant loss of glycemic control, and the favorable effects on blood lipids were still apparent.[46] Other studies have actually shown hemoglobin A_1C to drop, indicating improvement in blood sugar control.

The most common blood lipid abnormalities in type 2 diabetes patients are elevated triglyceride levels; decreased HDL levels; and a preponderance of smaller, denser LDL particles. Niacin has been shown to address all these areas much more significantly than statins and other lipid-lowering drugs.[44-46]

In addition to lowering cholesterol and triglycerides, niacin exerts additional benefits in battling atherosclerosis. Specifically, niacin produces beneficial lipid-altering effects on particle distribution in patients with coronary artery disease that are not well reflected in typical lipoprotein analysis. In addition, systemic markers of inflammation decrease in patients receiving niacin. In one study, when a modest dosage of niacin (1000 mg daily) was added to existing therapy for three months in 54 patients with stable coronary artery disease, there was a 32% increase in large-particle HDL, an 8% decrease in small-particle HDL, an 82% increase in large-particle LDL, and a 12% decrease in small-particle LDL.[47] Niacin therapy also decreased lipoprotein-associated phospholipase A2 and CRP levels (20% and 15%, respectively). No significant changes from baseline were seen in any tested parameter in patients who received a placebo.

These results indicate that the addition of niacin to existing medical regimens for patients with coronary artery disease and already well-controlled lipid levels favorably improves the distribution of lipoprotein particle sizes and inflammatory markers in a manner expected to improve protection against a cardiovascular event.

While niacin exerts significant benefit on its own, it does not appear to enhance the benefits of statins in well-controlled patients. The AIM-HIGH study funded by the National Heart, Lung, and Blood Institute recruited 3,400 patients who were at risk for heart trouble despite the fact that their LDL was under control with the use of a statin drug, simvastatin (Zocor). The study ended 18 months early because no additional cardiovascular benefit was seen in those taking niacin. Nonetheless, other studies are underway to determine the effect of niacin combined with a statin in patients with very low HDL levels and/or poorly controlled LDL levels.

SIDE EFFECTS OF NIACIN

The side effects of niacin are well known. The most common and bothersome side effect is the skin flushing that typically occurs 20–30 minutes after taking it. Other occasional side effects of niacin include gastric irritation, nausea, and liver damage. In an attempt to combat the acute reaction of skin flushing, several manufacturers began marketing sustained-release, timed-release, or slow-release niacin products. These formulations allow the niacin to be absorbed gradually, thereby reducing the flushing reaction.

However, although these forms of niacin reduce skin flushing, earlier timed-release preparations were proven to be more toxic to the liver than regular niacin. In one analysis, 52% of the patients taking the earlier sustained-release niacin preparations developed liver toxicity, while none of the patients taking immediate-release niacin developed liver toxicity.[48]

The newer timed-released preparations on the market, referred to as "intermediate-release," appear to have solved this problem, as relatively large clinical trials have shown them to be extremely well tolerated even when combined with statin drugs.[49-52] For example, the safety and tolerability of an intermediate-release niacin preparation was evaluated in a multicenter study of 566 patients.[52] The target dose was achieved by 65% of patients. Flushing was the most common side effect (42%), as expected, and 9.7% of patients withdrew because of flushing. Other drug-related adverse reactions occurred at low frequency (18.6%); 8.7% withdrew for adverse reactions other than flushing. Most adverse reactions were mild or moderate in severity. There were no liver toxicity or serious muscle adverse events.

Another safe form of niacin is inositol hexaniacinate. This form of niacin has long been used in Europe to lower cholesterol levels and to improve blood flow in a type of painful leg cramp known as intermittent claudication. It yields slightly better clinical results than standard niacin but is much better tolerated, in terms of both flushing and, more importantly, long-term side effects.[53,54]

Regardless of the form of niacin you choose, you need your doctor to periodically check (at a minimum, every three months) your cholesterol and liver function. Niacin should not be used in those with preexisting liver disease or elevation in liver enzymes. For these people, plant sterols, garlic, or pantethine are recommended.

For best results, niacin should be given at night, as most cholesterol synthesis occurs while sleeping. If pure crystalline niacin is being used, begin with a dose of 100 mg/day and carefully increase over 4–6 weeks to the full therapeutic dose of 1500–3000 mg daily. If a timed-released preparation (intermediate release only!) or inositol hexaniacinate is used, take a 500 mg dosage at night and increase to 1500 mg after two weeks. If after one month of therapy the dosage of 1500 mg per day fails to effectively lower LDL, increase the dosage to 2000 mg. If that dosage fails to lower lipids, increase the dosage to 3000 mg/day before discontinuing owing to lack of efficacy.

Typically, niacin (1000–2000 mg at night) reduces total cholesterol by 50–75 mg/dl in patients with initial total cholesterol levels above 250 mg/dl within the first two months. In patients with initial cholesterol levels above 300 mg/dl, it may take 4–6 months for cholesterol levels to begin to reach recommended levels. Once cholesterol levels are reduced below 200 mg/dl for two successive blood measurements at least two months apart, the dosage can be reduced for two months. If the cholesterol levels creep up above

200 mg/dl, then the dosage of niacin should be raised back up to previous levels. If the cholesterol level remains below 200 mg/dl, then the niacin can be withdrawn completely and the cholesterol levels rechecked in two months, with niacin therapy restarted if levels have exceeded 200 mg/dl. The same sort of schedule applies to other natural cholesterol-lowering agents.

SYTRINOL

A few years ago, a friend asked me if there were any natural alternatives to the statin drug Lipitor. His physician had prescribed the drug after a routine yearly physical showed that his cholesterol level was 294 mg/dl and his LDL level was 195 mg/dl. I told him there are many choices, but I wanted him to try a new product on the market, Sytrinol (a special flavonoid extract from citrus peels), combined with plant sterols. The research on Sytrinol is extremely impressive and I was looking for a test subject, so I asked my friend to take three capsules in the morning and three at night to provide a daily intake of 1200 mg of the plant sterols and 450 mg of Sytrinol.

His repeat blood test two months later showed that his total cholesterol had dropped to 190 mg/dl and his LDL was now 105 mg/dl. Both of these numbers are outstanding, representing a drop of more than 30% for the total cholesterol and roughly 45% for the LDL. Fantastic! It was just the response I had hoped for.

Clinical results have shown that Sytrinol exerts effects very similar to those of statin drugs, but without side effects.[55] Specifically, it has been shown to lower total cholesterol levels up to 30% and LDL levels up to 27%. But while statins do not lower triglyceride levels, Sytrinol is able to lower them by 34% within 4–12 weeks of use.

For best results, the recommended dosage is 150 mg of Sytrinol twice daily. For larger individuals and for people with total cholesterol levels over 300 mg/dl, I generally recommend 450 mg of Sytrinol daily.

PLANT STEROLS AND STANOLS

Phytosterols and phytostanols are structurally similar to cholesterol and can act in the intestine to lower cholesterol absorption by displacing cholesterol from intestinal micelles (an aggregate of water-insoluble molecules – like cholesterol – surrounded by water-soluble molecules, which facilitates absorption into the body). Because phytosterols and phytostanols are poorly absorbed themselves, blood cholesterol levels will drop owing to increased excretion. These compounds are showing up in functional foods (e.g., margarine and other spreads, orange juice), as well as in dietary supplements.

Phytosterols and phytostanols are effective in lowering LDL in some people. A meta-analysis of 41 trials showed that a daily intake of 2000 mg of stanols or sterols reduces LDL by 10%.[56] Taking higher dosages added little additional benefit. The effects of phytosterols and phytostanols are additive with diet or drug interventions: Eating foods low in saturated fat and cholesterol and high in stanols or sterols can reduce LDL by 20%; adding sterols or stanols to statin medication is more effective than doubling the statin dose alone. Individuals most likely to respond have been identified as having high cholesterol absorption and low cholesterol biosynthesis. Phytosterols and phytostanols have also shown antiplatelet and antioxidant effects.[57–59]

Be aware, however, that phytosterol or phytostanol intake at higher dosages may reduce carotenoid absorption. People consuming 6600 mg/day of phytosterols showed cholesterol-adjusted plasma reduction of alpha and beta carotene levels (down 19–23%), lutein (14%), and lycopene (11%). This effect was partially reversed by increased fruit and vegetable intake.[60]

PANTETHINE

Pantethine is the stable form of pantetheine, the active form of vitamin B5, or pantothenic acid. Pantothenic acid is the most important component of coenzyme A (CoA). This enzyme is involved in the transport of fats to and from cells, as well as to the energy-producing compartments within the cell. Without coenzyme A, the cell's fats cannot be metabolized to energy.

Pantethine has significant lipid-lowering activity while pantothenic acid has little (if any) effect in lowering cholesterol and triglyceride levels, owing to pantethine's ability to be converted to cysteamine. Pantethine administration (standard dose 900 mg/day) has been shown to significantly reduce serum triglycerides (by 32%), total cholesterol (19%), and LDL (21%) levels while increasing HDL (23%) levels.[61,62] It appears to be especially useful in diabetics.[63-65]

The lipid-lowering effects of pantethine are most impressive when its toxicity (virtually none) is compared with that of conventional lipid-lowering drugs. Its mechanism of action is due to inhibited cholesterol synthesis and acceleration of the use of fat as an energy source.

GARLIC *(ALLIUM SATIVUM)* AND ONION *(ALLIUM CEPA)*

Garlic appears to be an important protective factor against heart disease and stroke owing to its ability to affect the process of atherosclerosis at so many steps. A major area of focus on garlic's ability to offer significant protection against heart disease and strokes has been the evaluation of its ability to lower blood cholesterol levels, even in apparently healthy individuals. According to the results from numerous double-blind, placebo-controlled studies in patients with initial cholesterol levels greater than 200 mg/dl, supplementation with commercial preparations providing a daily dose of at least 10 mg alliin or a total allicin potential of 4000 mcg can lower total serum cholesterol by about 10–12%; LDL decreases by about 15%, HDL usually increases by about 10%, and triglycerides typically drop by 15%. However, most trials not using products that can deliver this dosage of allicin fail to show a lipid-lowering effect.[66-70]

Although the effects of supplemental garlic preparations on cholesterol levels are modest, the combination of lowering LDL and raising HDL can greatly improve the HDL:LDL ratio, a significant goal in the prevention of heart disease and strokes. Garlic preparations have also demonstrated blood pressure lowering effects; inhibition of platelet aggregation; reduction of plasma viscosity; promotion of fibrinolysis; prevention of LDL oxidation; and an ability to exert positive effects on endothelial function, vascular re-activity, and peripheral blood flow.

Table 3.6 Comparative Effects on Blood Lipids of Several Natural Compounds

Effect	Niacin	Garlic	Pantethine
Total cholesterol (% decrease)	18	10	19
LDL cholesterol (% decrease)	23	15	21
HDL cholesterol (% increase)	32	31	23
Triglycerides (% decrease)	26	13	32

FINAL COMMENTS

I recognize that this chapter is probably a bit overwhelming and may be in direct conflict with the recommendations of your physician. Here are some key takeaway points:

- Statins are largely prescribed based on misinformation the doctor has received from the drug companies and their representatives.

- Niacin is a suitable alternative to a statin and can be a compromise, although the research shows niacin produces the best overall effect.

- Consuming a diet rich in cholesterol-lowering factors can produce the same level of cholesterol reduction as a lower dosage of a statin.

- Keep in mind that cholesterol levels are just one piece of the puzzle of reducing cardiovascular disease.

- Though fish oils do not usually affect cholesterol levels, they do lower triglycerides and produce benefits that far exceed their effect on blood lipids.

If you are still confused and wondering what to do, here's what I recommend:

- Do everything you can to get your cholesterol levels in the ideal range without taking a statin drug first. Follow the dietary recommendations above. In cases where the initial total cholesterol level is above 300 mg/dl or LDL is greater than 170 mg/dl, I recommend taking a combination of Sytrinol (150 mg twice daily) and niacin (2000 mg daily). If the numbers are lower, then take either niacin or Sytrinol and repeat blood tests every two months.

- If you have an HDL level of less than 50 mg/dl, then take 2000 mg of niacin at night, a garlic product providing a daily dose of at least 10 mg alliin or a total allicin potential of 4000 mcg, and get more exercise.

- If you are currently taking a statin drug or red yeast rice and your cholesterol levels are in the recommended range, I would recommend working with your doctor and starting the dietary recommendations and the combination of niacin and Sytrinol. After 4–6 weeks, reduce the statin dosage by half. It is very important to recheck the cholesterol levels 4–6 weeks after reducing the statin dosage. If everything looks great, try eliminating the statin entirely and recheck again in 4–6 weeks.

- If your cholesterol levels are not in the ideal range even though you are on a statin, I would definitely recommend adding niacin to your regimen. Continue to monitor your cholesterol levels with your doctor.

- If you must take a statin because it is medically indicated in your case (please see discussion above), then you must absolutely supplement your diet with 200 mg of CoQ_{10} daily.

- If you have high triglycerides, take a high-quality fish oil supplement at a dosage that will deliver 3000 mg of EPA+DHA (combined) per day.

Also, keep in mind that regular physical exercise is extremely important in reducing the risk of heart disease and strokes. It accomplishes this goal by lowering cholesterol levels, improving blood and oxygen supply to the heart, increasing the functional capacity of the heart, reducing blood pressure, reducing obesity, and exerting a favorable effect on blood clotting.

CHAPTER 4

BEYOND CHOLESTEROL: THE ROLE OF INSULIN RESISTANCE

In Chapter 1, I stated that a strong argument could be made that insulin resistance is much more important than elevated cholesterol levels as a risk factor for atherosclerosis (hardening of the arteries) and cardiovascular disease (CVD). In fact, if we look at the big picture it's easy to conclude that insulin resistance is the biggest factor contributing to an increased risk of heart disease in most North Americans.

Insulin resistance means that your body becomes less sensitive to the actions of your own insulin. One of the key actions of insulin is to drive glucose from blood into the cells. Insulin resistance promotes atherosclerosis and CVD by the following mechanisms:

- Elevated blood sugar levels are associated with increased attachment of glucose to receptor proteins, leading to loss of key feedback mechanisms. For example, if the receptor for low-density lipoprotein cholesterol (LDL; "bad" cholesterol) on the surface of a liver cell becomes damaged by the attachment of glucose, the liver cell does not get the feedback message that there is plenty of cholesterol. In fact, without the feedback the liver cell thinks it needs to make more cholesterol.

- Elevated levels of blood sugar are also associated with increased oxidative stress leading to damage to LDL, as well as adding fuel to the fire of silent inflammation. In fact, insulin resistance is the key factor in causing silent inflammation and high levels of high-sensitivity C-reactive protein (hsCRP). Much of the inflammatory effect of insulin resistance is due to its negative effects on the endothelium, the lining of the blood vessel wall.

- Since there is a relative deficiency of glucose within cells because of insulin resistance, even though blood sugar levels are high, the pancreas begins dumping larger quantities of insulin into the blood. Higher blood insulin levels are now a well-established risk factor for heart disease. A high level of insulin in the blood promotes atherosclerosis by several mechanisms, including stimulating smooth muscle cell proliferation in the arterial wall, leading to thickening and stiffness of the arterial wall as well as narrowing of the artery.

- Insulin resistance is associated with high blood pressure. It not only contributes to more rigid and constricted blood vessels, it causes retention of sodium and water from the kidneys, which then leads to high blood pressure.

- Insulin resistance promotes greater fat breakdown, leading to the characteristic blood lipid pattern of elevated LDL and triglycerides with lower levels of high-density lipoprotein cholesterol (HDL; "good" cholesterol). In normal individuals, one of the functions of insulin is to suppress the breakdown of fat from the fat cells into the bloodstream. With insulin resistance this effect is blocked, leading to an exaggerated breakdown of fat from the fat cells and the release of free fatty acids into the blood. The liver takes up these free fatty acids and converts them into triglycerides in the form of very-low-density lipoprotein (VLDL), which ultimately lowers HDL levels. Insulin resistance also increases the formation of the smaller, more dense LDL.

- Insulin resistance increases platelet aggregation and fibrinogen levels. This scenario greatly increases the risk for clot formation. In addition, insulin resistance blocks the action of tissue plasminogen activator, a clot-busting compound produced by the cells that line the artery.

- Insulin resistance is associated with increased levels of the adrenal hormone cortisol.

WHAT CAUSES INSULIN RESISTANCE?

Insulin resistance is tied to abdominal obesity. If your waist circumference is larger than your hips, there is an extremely strong likelihood that you suffer from insulin resistance. As fat cells in the abdomen grow in size or number, they secrete a number of biologic products (e.g., resistin) that dampen the effect of insulin, impair glucose utilization in skeletal muscle, and promote glucose (blood sugar) production by the liver. Also important is that as the number and size of fat cells increase, they lead to a reduction in the secretion of compounds that promote insulin action, including a novel protein produced by fat cells known as adiponectin.

Adiponectin is not only associated with improved insulin sensitivity, it also has anti-inflammatory activity, lowers triglycerides, and blocks the development of atherosclerosis. The net effect of all these actions by fat cells in the overweight individual is that they severely stress blood sugar control mechanisms and lead to the development of the major complication of diabetes – atherosclerosis. Because of all these newly discovered hormones secreted by fat cells, the collective fatty tissue in the body is considered part of the hormonal (endocrine) system.

HOW BIG IS THE PROBLEM?

If you are overweight you are definitely not alone. Current estimates are that eight out of 10 adults in the United States are overweight, with about half of these people, 40% of our adult population, meeting the criteria for obesity. It's a huge issue that is crippling our health care systems and our productivity. Each year obesity-related conditions cost over $100 billion and cause an estimated 300,000 premature deaths in the U.S., making a very strong case that the obesity epidemic is the most significant threat to the future of the United States, as well as other nations.

In addition to the epidemic of obesity there is a parallel epidemic of type 2 diabetes. Currently, 20 million Americans meet the criteria for type 2 diabetes and another 80 million suffer from prediabetes – a condition characterized by insulin resistance – and/or metabolic syndrome. All told, over 100 million people in the United States show signs of significant insulin resistance.

OBESITY AND MORTALITY

Obese individuals have an average life expectancy 5–7 years shorter than that of normal-weight individuals, with a greater relative risk for mortality associated with a greater degree of obesity.[1,2] Most of the increased risk for mortality is due to CVD, because obesity carries with it a tremendous risk for type 2 diabetes, elevated cholesterol levels, high blood pressure, and other risk factors for atherosclerosis. In 2009 the annual medical spending due to overweight and obesity was estimated to be $147 billion.[3]

HOW DO YOU KNOW IF YOU HAVE INSULIN RESISTANCE?

One of the most useful clinical determinants of insulin resistance is simply measuring the waist to hip ratio. However, if the waist circumference for a man is greater than 40 inches, and for a woman greater than 30 inches, there is no need to do any further calculation because this measurement alone has been shown to be a major risk factor for both CVD and type 2 diabetes, two of the biggest consequences of insulin resistance, as well as high blood pressure and gout. A waist to hip ratio above 1.0 for men and above 0.8 for women is highly predictive of insulin resistance. To determine your waist to hip ratio,

1. Measure the circumference of your waist: _____

2. Measure the circumference of your hips: _____

3. Divide the waist measurement by the hip measurement: waist/hip = _____ . This is your waist/hip ratio.

IMPROVING INSULIN SENSITIVITY

Improving blood sugar control, whether the goal is weight loss, reduction of risk factors for CVD, or prevention of type 2 diabetes, is most successfully done with a combination of lifestyle changes, such as increasing physical activity and improving diet and nutrition, and targeted nutritional supplementation.

Obviously, dietary carbohydrates play a central role in the cause, prevention, and treatment of insulin resistance and type 2 diabetes. In an effort to label carbohydrate sources as good or bad, one useful tool is the glycemic index (GI). It is a numerical scale used to indicate how fast and how high a particular food raises blood glucose levels compared with glucose. Refined sugars, white flour products, and other sources of simple sugars are quickly absorbed into the bloodstream, causing a rapid rise in blood sugar, severely stressing blood sugar control. So it is important to avoid junk food and pay attention to the GI of the food you eat.

Studies have shown that an elevated after-meal blood sugar level is a greater risk factor for heart disease that abnormal fasting plasma glucose.[4,5] So even if you do not have insulin resistance it is critical to avoid high blood sugar levels at any time to prevent CVD.

Table 4.1 Classification of Foods by Glycemic Index Scores

Fruits and Nonstarchy Vegetables			
Very High	**High**	**Medium**	**Low**
None	Bananas	Cantaloupe	Apples
	Raisins	Grapes	Apricots
	Beets	Oranges	Asparagus
		Orange juice	Broccoli
		Peaches	Brussels sprouts
		Pineapples	Cauliflower
		Watermelon	Celery
			Cherries
			Cucumbers
			Grapefruit
			Green beans
			Green peppers
			Lettuce
			Mushrooms
			Onions
			Plums
			Spinach
			Strawberries
			Tomatoes
			Zucchini

Grains, Nuts, Legumes, and Starchy Vegetables			
Very High	**High**	**Medium**	**Low**
Refined sugar and flour products	Bagels	Bread (rye)	Lentils
Most cold cereals (e.g., Grape-Nuts, corn flakes, Raisin Bran, etc.)	Bread (white)	Bread (whole-grain)	Nuts
Rice cakes	Carrots	Brown rice	Seeds
Granola	Corn	Oatmeal	
	Granola bars	Pasta	
	Kidney beans	Peas	
	Muffins (bran)	Pita bread	
	Potatoes	Pinto beans	
	Pretzels	Yams	
	White rice		
	Tortillas		

The GI is quite useful, but since it doesn't tell you how much carbohydrate is in a typical serving of a particular food, another tool is needed. That is where glycemic load comes in. The glycemic load (GL) is a relatively new way to assess the impact of carbohydrate consumption. It takes the glycemic index into account, but gives a more complete picture of the effect that a particular food has on blood sugar levels based on how much carbohydrate you actually eat in a serving. A GL of 20 or more is high, a GL of 11–19 inclusive is medium, and a GL of 10 or less is low.

For example, let's take a look at beets, a food with a high GI, but low GL. Although the carbohydrate in beets has a high GI, there isn't a lot of it, so a typical serving of cooked beets has a very low GL, about 5. Thus, as long as you eat a reasonable portion of a low-glycemic-load food, the impact on blood sugar is acceptable, even if the food has a high GI.

Table 4.2 Examples of Glycemic Index, Glycemic Load, and Insulin Stress Scores of Selected Foods

Food	Glycemic Index	Glycemic Load	Insulin Stress (Glycemic Impact)
Carrots, cooked, ½ cup	49	1.5	Low
Peach, fresh, 1 large	42	3.0	Low
Beets, cooked ½ cup	64	3.0	Low
Watermelon, ½ cup	72	4.0	Low
Bread, whole-wheat, 1 slice	69	9.6	Low
Potato, baked, medium	93	14.0	Medium
Rice, brown, cooked, 1 cup	50	16.0	Medium
Banana, raw, 1 medium	55	17.6	Medium
Spaghetti, white, cooked, 1 cup	41	23.0	High
Rice, white, cooked, 1 cup	72	26.0	High
Grape-Nuts cereal, ½ cup	71	33.0	Very high
Soft drinks, 375 ml	68	34.7	Very high

To help you design your diet, I have provided a list of the GI, fiber content, and GL of common foods in Appendix B. In essence, foods that are mostly water (e.g., apple or watermelon), fiber (e.g., beet root or carrot), or air (e.g., popcorn) will not cause a steep rise in your blood sugar even if their GI is high, as long as you exercise moderation in portion sizes. I recommend keeping the GL for any three-hour period to less than 20.

THE IMPORTANCE OF DIETARY FIBER IN IMPROVING INSULIN SENSITIVITY

Population studies, as well as clinical and experimental data, show diabetes to be one of the diseases most clearly related to inadequate dietary fiber intake. Different types of fibers possess different actions. The type of fiber that exerts the most beneficial effects on blood sugar control is the water-soluble form. Included in this class are hemicelluloses, mucilages, gums, and pectin substances. These types of fiber are capable of slowing down the digestion and absorption of carbohydrates, thereby preventing rapid rises in blood sugar. These fibers are also associated with increasing the sensitivity of tissues to insulin and improving the uptake of glucose by the muscles, liver, and other tissues, thereby preventing a sustained elevation of blood sugar.[6,7]

Particularly good sources of water-soluble fiber are legumes, oat bran, nuts, seeds, psyllium seed husks, pears, apples, and most vegetables. Large amounts of plant foods must be consumed to obtain enough dietary fiber, although beans, peas, and legumes are overall the best sources for high fiber intake in relatively easy amounts to ingest.

Although even the simple change from white-flour products to whole-grain versions is associated with a reduced risk for type 2 diabetes,[8,9] my recommendation is to consume at least 35 g of fiber a day from various food sources, especially vegetables. For people with insulin resistance, it is critical to take PGX® at all meals to reduce after-meal elevations in blood sugar levels. Human clinical trials with PGX® have shown it to have an impressive effect in reducing the glycemic impact of any food or meal.[10–12]

PGX® IS A KEY TOOL FOR IMPROVING INSULIN SENSITIVITY

PGX® (short for PolyGlycopleX ®) is a completely new and unique fiber matrix. The effectiveness of any fiber on reducing appetite, blood sugar, and cholesterol is based directly on the amount of water the fiber is able to absorb and the degree of thickness or viscosity the fiber imparts when in the stomach and intestine. For instance, this water solubility and viscosity is why oat bran lowers cholesterol and controls blood sugar better gram for gram than wheat bran. With this in mind, researchers have been seeking to identify and isolate dietary fibers with the highest viscosity and water-holding capacity in order to make them available as food ingredients or nutritional supplements.

DIETARY FAT AND INSULIN RESISTANCE

Dietary fat also plays a central role in insulin sensitivity. The type of dietary fat profile linked to insulin resistance is an abundance of saturated fat from animal foods and trans fatty acids (partially hydrogenated vegetable oils) along with a relative insufficiency of monounsaturated and omega-3 fatty acids. One of the key reasons appears to be the fact that because dietary fat determines cell membrane composition, such a dietary pattern leads to reduced membrane fluidity, which in turn causes reduced insulin binding to receptors on cellular membranes or reduced insulin action, or both.[13]

Particularly harmful to cell membrane function are margarine, vegetable oil shortening, and other foods containing trans fatty acids and partially hydrogenated oils. These fatty acids interfere with the body's ability to use important essential fatty acids. One study estimated that substituting polyunsaturated vegetable oils for margarine that contains partially hydrogenated vegetable oil would reduce the likelihood of developing type 2 diabetes by 40%.[14]

In contrast to the dampening of insulin sensitivity caused by partially hydrogenated margarine and saturated fats, clinical studies have shown that monounsaturated fats and omega-3 oils improve insulin action.[15] Adding further support is the fact that population studies have also indicated that frequent consumption of monounsaturated fats such as olive oil, raw or lightly roasted nuts and seeds, nut oils, and omega-3 fatty acids from fish protect against the development of type 2 diabetes. Healthy omega-3 fish include wild salmon, trout, anchovies, sardines, halibut, and herring. All of this evidence clearly indicates that altered cell membrane composition and fluidity play a critical role in the development of type 2 diabetes.

One of the most useful foods to reduce the risk of type 2 diabetes is nuts. Studies have shown that consumption of nuts is inversely associated with risk of type 2 diabetes, independent of known risk factors, including age, obesity, family history of diabetes, physical inactivity, smoking, and other dietary factors.[16] In addition to providing beneficial monounsaturated and polyunsaturated fats that improve insulin sensitivity, nuts are also rich in fiber and magnesium and have a low GI. Higher intakes of fiber and magnesium and foods with a low GI have been associated with reduced risk of type 2 diabetes in several population-based studies. Eating mostly raw or lightly roasted fresh nuts and seeds rather than commercially roasted and salted nuts and seeds is advocated.

Through a special process, natural fibers are transformed to make PGX® the most viscous and soluble fiber ever discovered. What that means is that all the health benefits linked to soluble dietary fiber – including stabilizing blood sugar levels – are significantly magnified with PGX®. Detailed analysis has shown that PGX® produces a higher level of viscosity, gel-forming properties, and expansion with water than the same quantity of any other fiber alone.

The PGX® matrix is able to bind hundreds of times its weight in water, resulting in a volume and viscosity 3–5 times greater than that of other highly soluble fibers such as psyllium or oat beta glucan. To put this in perspective, a small 5 g serving of PGX® in a meal replacement formula or on its own produces a volume and viscosity that would be equal to as much as four bowls of oat bran. In this way, small quantities of PGX® can be added to foods or taken as a drink before meals to have an impact on appetite and blood sugar control equivalent to eating enormous and impractical quantities of any other form of fiber.

Detailed clinical studies published in major medical journals and presented at the world's major diabetes conferences have shown PGX® to exert the following benefits:[10–12,16–18]

- Stabilizes blood sugar in the overweight and obese
- Reduces appetite and promotes effective weight loss, even in the morbidly obese
- Increases the level of compounds that block the appetite and promote satiety
- Decreases the level of compounds that stimulate overeating
- Reduces after-meal blood glucose levels when added to or taken with food
- Reduces the GI of any food or beverage
- Increases insulin sensitivity and decreases blood insulin
- Improves diabetes control and dramatically reduces the need for medications or insulin in diabetics
- Lowers blood cholesterol and triglycerides

PGX® REDUCES BLOOD SUGAR VOLATILITY

By using new techniques in 24-hour blood sugar monitoring, ground-breaking research conducted by Michael Lyon, MD, and others at the Canadian Centre for Functional Medicine has shown that excessive appetite and food cravings in overweight people are directly correlated with rapid fluctuations in blood glucose throughout the day and night. Furthermore, it has now been documented that by using PGX®, these same patients can dramatically restore their body's ability to tightly control blood sugar levels and that this accomplishment is powerfully linked to remarkable improvements in blood sugar control, reductions in appetite, and safe and effective weight loss.

Figure 4.1 is an example of what this data looks like before beginning the PGX® weight loss program. Figure 4.2 shows the data after four weeks of the program.

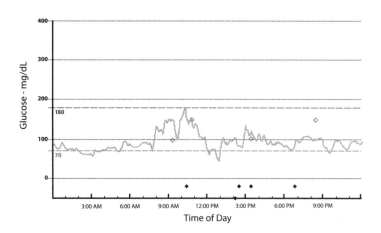

Figure 4.1 Continuous glucose graph over 24 hours in typical overweight, nondiabetic patient before beginning the PGX® program. Patient has elevated glycemic volatility (she is on the "blood sugar roller coaster"). Monitoring for several days showed that this was her consistent pattern even when she ate healthy food. Frequent food cravings were reported at times when blood sugar rapidly dropped over short periods. This amounted to several significant food cravings per day. Feelings of hypoglycemia also occurred when blood sugar dropped rapidly, even when blood sugar was above the normal range (i.e., 70–100 mg/dl). This patient was spending most of the day outside this ideal range.

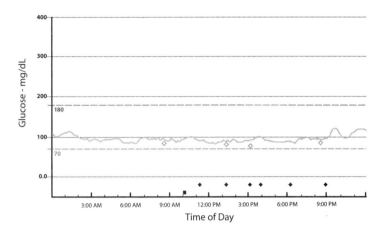

Figure 4.2 Continuous glucose graph over 24 hours in same patient four weeks into the PGX® program. Patient now has nearly normalized glycemic volatility. Appetite and food cravings have dramatically diminished. Hypoglycemic symptoms no longer occur. As well, patient has more energy and mental clarity. Weight loss is progressing on target and with no discomfort. This type of change is typical with PGX® use and it dramatically illustrates the remarkable changes that can occur.

HOW TO USE PGX®

PGX® works best if it is used with a low-glycemic diet (discussed below). The dosage of PGX® is based on your needs. If you don't need to lose weight and simply want to take advantage of the ability of PGX® to stabilize blood sugar levels, the dosage is only 750–1500 mg before meals. However, if you want to lose weight, then the dosage needs to be at least 2500–5000 mg before meals (start with a dosage of 750–1000 mg and work your way up to the full dosage over the course of a couple of weeks).

PGX® is available in a variety of different forms: soft gelatin capsules, a zero-calorie drink mix, granules to be added to food and beverages, and a meal replacement drink mix containing undenatured whey protein, natural flavors, and sweeteners along with vitamins and minerals (SlimStyles Weight Loss Drink). It does not matter which form you use, just make sure you get the required dosage of PGX® before each meal. For weight loss, I like to recommend taking another dose of PGX® about an hour after dinner to reduce nighttime eating. Be sure to drink 8 oz of water for each 2500 mg dose. For many people, taking PGX® in soft gelatin capsules 5–15 minutes before meals with a glass of water is the most convenient way to use PGX®.

Detailed studies in both humans and animals have shown that PGX® is very safe and well tolerated. There are no specific drug interactions, but it is best to take any medication either an hour before or after taking PGX®.

For more information see pgx.com. Appendix C also provides answers to some of the common questions about PGX®.

FINAL COMMENTS

Here are my concise recommendations for individuals with insulin resistance, prediabetes, or type 2 diabetes. Keep in mind that it's important to recognize that as the natural therapies described in this chapter take effect, drug dosages may need to be altered and that a good working relationship with the prescribing doctor is required. The ultimate goal is to re-establish normal blood sugar control without drugs and prevent the development of the complications of diabetes, including CVD – CVD is the cause of death in 55% of diabetics.

DIET

Start each meal by taking PGX® at a dosage of 2500–5000 mg. It's important to follow the dietary guidelines detailed in Chapter 2. All simple, processed, concentrated carbohydrates must be avoided. A low-glycemic diet rich in high-fiber foods should be stressed, and sources of healthy fats should be ingested. Low-glycemic vegetables, onions, and garlic are particularly useful and their liberal consumption is encouraged.

NUTRITIONAL SUPPLEMENTS FOR PREDIABETES AND TYPE 2 DIABETES

The recommended supplementation program depends on the degree of blood glucose control, as shown by self-monitored blood glucose and A_1C levels.

LEVEL 1 – ACHIEVEMENT OF TARGETED BLOOD GLUCOSE AND A₁C LEVELS LESS THAN 7%, NO LIPID ABNORMALITIES, NO SIGNS OF COMPLICATIONS:

- High-potency multivitamin and mineral
- Fish oils: 1000 mg of EPA+DHA daily
- Vitamin C: 500–1500 mg daily
- Vitamin E: 400–800 IU daily (mixed tocopherols)
- Grape seed, pine bark, or green tea extract (or other appropriate flavonoid-rich extract): 100–150 mg daily
- Alpha-lipoic acid: 400–600 mg daily

LEVEL 2 – FAILURE TO ACHIEVE TARGETED BLOOD GLUCOSE LEVELS, A₁C ABOVE 7%; LEVEL 1 SUPPORT PLUS:

- Insulin enhancer – use one of the following:
  - *G. sylvestre* extract (24% gymnemic acid): 200 mg twice daily
  - Fenugreek extract: 1000 mg daily
  - Garlic: minimum 4000 mcg of allicin daily
- Mulberry extract: equivalent to 1000 mg dried leaf three times daily

If self-monitored blood glucose levels do not improve after four weeks of following the recommendations for the current level, move to the next level. For example, if a person starts out having an A₁C level of 8.2% and a fasting blood glucose level of 130 mg/dl, he or she should start on Level 2 support. After four weeks, if the average reading has not dropped to less than 110 mg/dl, then a prescription medication (either an oral hypoglycemic drug or insulin) is required.

FOR HIGH CHOLESTEROL LEVELS

For high cholesterol levels and other cardiovascular risk factors (total cholesterol greater than 200 mg/dl or LDL greater than 135 mg/dl, 100 mg/dl if there is a history of heart attack); HDL below 45 mg/dl; lipoprotein(a) above 40 mg/dl; or triglycerides above 150 mg/dl:

- Niacin: 1000–2000 mg at bedtime
- Garlic: minimum of 4000 mcg of allicin daily

FOR HIGH BLOOD PRESSURE

- Garlic: minimum of 4000 mcg of allicin daily
- Coenzyme Q_{10}: 200 mg daily
- Anti-ACE peptides from bonito: 1500 mg daily
- Take one of the following:

  · Hawthorn extract (10% procyanidins or 1.8% vitexin-4'-rhamnoside): 100–250 mg three times daily

  · Olive leaf extract (17–23% oleuropein content): 500 mg twice daily

  · Hibiscus: three 240 ml servings per day or an extract providing 10–20 mg anthocyanidins daily

CHAPTER 5

THE HEART HEALTHY LIFESTYLE

Without question, a healthy lifestyle improves the quality and length of life. It's mostly common sense – develop positive relationships, avoid harmful habits like smoking and drinking excessively, get a good night's sleep, and exercise. Many of these key components of a heart healthy lifestyle were briefly mentioned in Chapter 1. In particular, the tremendously deadly effects of cigarette smoking were pointed out. The importance of exercise and avoiding the expression of hostility and anger were also mentioned.

I want to start this chapter off by once again highlighting the fact that individuals with type A behavior (e.g., extreme sense of time urgency, competitiveness, impatience, and aggressiveness) have a twofold increase in cardiovascular disease (CVD) over non-type A individuals. Particularly damaging to the cardiovascular system is the expression of negative emotions and anger. Greater expression of anger is associated with a lower ratio of low-density lipoprotein (LDL) to high-density lipoprotein (HDL), increased high-sensitivity C-reactive protein (hsCRP), increased secretion of stress hormones such as cortisol, dysfunction in the lining of the arteries, high blood pressure, and excessive blood clot formation.[1-3]

The bottom line from all this research is that expression of hostility and anger comes back to cause harm to the individual expressing it as well as the victims it leaves in its wake. Here are 10 tips to improve your coping strategies and reduce your feelings of anger and hostility:

1. **DO NOT STARVE YOUR EMOTIONAL LIFE.** Foster meaningful relationships. Make time to give and receive love in your life.

2. **LEARN TO BE A GOOD LISTENER.** Allow the people in your life to really share their feelings and thoughts uninterrupted. Empathize with them; put yourself in their shoes.

3. **DO NOT TRY TO TALK OVER OTHERS.** If you find yourself being interrupted, relax; do not try to outtalk the other person. If you are courteous and allow other people to speak, eventually (unless they are extremely rude) they will reciprocate. If not, explain that they are disrupting the communication process. You can do this only if you have been a good listener.

4. **AVOID AGGRESSIVE OR PASSIVE BEHAVIOR.** Be assertive, but express your thoughts and feelings in a kind way to help improve relationships at work and at home.

5. **AVOID EXCESSIVE STRESS IN YOUR LIFE AS BEST YOU CAN** by avoiding excessive work hours, poor nutrition, and inadequate rest. Get as much sleep as you can.

6. **AVOID STIMULANTS SUCH AS CAFFEINE AND NICOTINE.** Stimulants promote the fight-or-flight response and tend to make people more irritable in the process.

7. **TAKE TIME TO BUILD LONG-TERM HEALTH AND SUCCESS** by performing stress-reduction techniques and deep breathing exercises.

8. **ACCEPT GRACEFULLY THOSE THINGS OVER WHICH YOU HAVE NO CONTROL.** Save your energy for those things you can do something about.

9. **ACCEPT YOURSELF.** Remember that you are human and will make mistakes from which you can learn along the way.

10. **BE MORE PATIENT AND TOLERANT OF OTHER PEOPLE.** Follow the Golden Rule.

FROM GRIZZLY BEAR TO TEDDY BEAR

My favorite example of the healing power of a merry heart is Jerry. At the time of his first visit to me he was a 52-year-old United States Postal Service employee on medical disability leave. In the 11 years since he'd turned 41, Jerry had undergone seven heart surgeries – three coronary artery bypass operations and four angioplasties. Despite all these procedures and all the drugs he was taking, Jerry had tremendous angina with even the slightest exertion. The first time I saw him, in fact, he had an angina attack just walking the few feet from the waiting room to my office. He quickly popped a nitroglycerine pill; it was just one of the 11 prescription drugs he was taking, some of which were designed to reduce the side effects of other drugs.

Jerry was suffering from a severe case of heart failure – these medications were necessary to keep his weakened heart beating well enough to keep him alive. Jerry's heart disease was so severe that he was on the list for a heart transplant. What was an extremely fascinating feature in Jerry's case was that he had no risk factors identifiable by conventional testing. His cholesterol levels were perfect, his blood pressure was actually low, he did not smoke, and he was not overweight. For years, his doctors had been at a loss to explain why he had such severe heart disease.

It didn't take long for me to figure it out. Jerry seemed like a very affable, mild-mannered guy. But when I asked him how he would evaluate his ability to control his temper I could see that he often "went postal." I found it ironic that he was a postal worker. He told me he was a real hothead and that his temper was a major problem in his life. I once made the mistake of asking him to give me some examples of what made him mad. His face turned red, the veins in his neck and forehead popped out, and his voice became quite loud as he told me a few things that really ticked him off. Shortly into this tirade he stopped for a second or two to pop another nitroglycerin pill.

At that point, I seized the opportunity to help him make the connection between his inability to control his anger and his heart disease. He was quite resistant at first, because he just wanted me to prescribe some natural medicines. While I did provide him with a supplement regimen, I knew that the real key to getting Jerry better was for him to take a look at his emotional life. It did not happen all at once, but over the next few visits he really opened up and became receptive to my ideas. One of my initial prescriptions to Jerry was to read a book by my friend, noted cardiologist Dr. Stephen T. Sinatra: *Heartbreak and Heart Disease: A Mind/Body Prescription for Healing the Heart.* It is an excellent account of the role emotions play in heart disease. I also referred Jerry to a psychotherapist for biofeedback training and to a yoga instructor so he could start taking yoga classes.

Within two years from when I first saw Jerry, he went from popping nitroglycerin tablets practically every time he got up out of his chair to walking nearly four miles per day. His heart function went from less than 20% of normal, despite being on a long list of drugs, to nearly 80% of normal without any prescription medicines at all. Even more impressive than the improvements in his physical health were the changes in his emotional health and personality. What impressed me most, in fact, was the change in Jerry's relationship with his wife and kids.

So what led to the improvement? Was it the natural medicines I prescribed Jerry, or the changes he made in his emotional responses? No doubt the natural medicines improved his physical well-being. But I am convinced that the most important factor in Jerry's remarkable case was the emotional changes he made. By making those changes Jerry eliminated the major obstacle to wellness in his life.

LEARNING TO CALM THE MIND

An important step in fighting stress is learning to calm the mind and body. Relaxation exercises are among the easiest methods to learn. The goal of relaxation techniques is to produce a physiologic response known as the "relaxation response" – a response that is exactly opposite to the stress response and that reflects activation of the parasympathetic nervous system. Although an individual may relax by simply sleeping, watching television, or reading a book, relaxation techniques are designed specifically to produce the relaxation response.

Relaxation response is a term coined by Harvard professor and cardiologist Herbert Benson in the early 1970s to describe a physiologic response he found in people who meditate that is just the opposite of the stress response.[4] With the stress response, the sympathetic nervous system dominates to produce the fight-or-flight response. With the relaxation response, the parasympathetic nervous system dominates. The parasympathetic nervous system controls bodily functions such as digestion, breathing, and heart rate during periods of rest, relaxation, visualization, meditation, and sleep. The sympathetic nervous system is designed to protect against immediate danger; the parasympathetic system is designed for repair, maintenance, and restoration of the body.

The relaxation response can be achieved through a variety of techniques. It doesn't matter which technique you choose, because all techniques have the same physiologic effect – a state of deep relaxation. The most popular techniques are meditation, prayer, progressive relaxation, self-hypnosis, and biofeedback. To produce the desired long-term health benefits, you should use the relaxation technique for at least 5–10 minutes each day.

The relaxation response entails the following:

- The heart rate is reduced and the heart beats more effectively. Blood pressure is reduced.

- Blood is shunted toward internal organs, especially those organs involved in digestion.

- The rate of breathing decreases – oxygen demand is reduced during periods of rest.

- Sweat production diminishes, because a person who is calm and relaxed does not experience nervous perspiration.

- Production of digestive secretions is increased, greatly improving digestion.

- Blood sugar levels are maintained in the normal physiologic range.

LEARNING TO BREATHE

Producing deep relaxation with any relaxation technique requires learning how to breathe. Have you ever noticed how a baby breathes? With each breath the baby's abdomen rises and falls because the baby is breathing with its diaphragm, a dome-shaped muscle that separates the chest cavity from the abdominal cavity. If you are like most adults, you tend to fill only your upper chest because you do not use the diaphragm. Shallow breathing tends to produce tension and fatigue.

One of the most powerful methods of producing less stress and more energy in the body is by breathing with the diaphragm. By using the diaphragm to breath, a person dramatically changes their physiology. It literally activates the relaxation centers in the brain.

Here is a 10-step technique for learning diaphragmatic breathing.

1. Find a comfortable, quiet place to lie down or sit.

2. Place your feet slightly apart. Place one hand on your abdomen near your navel. Place the other hand on your chest.

3. You will be inhaling through your nose and exhaling through your mouth.

4. Concentrate on your breathing. Note which hand is rising and falling with each breath.

5. Gently exhale most of the air in your lungs.

6. Inhale while slowly counting to four. As you inhale, slightly extend your abdomen, causing it to rise about one inch. Make sure you are not moving your chest or shoulders.

7. As you breathe in, imagine the warmed air flowing in. Imagine this warmth flowing to all parts of your body.

8. Pause for one second, then slowly exhale to a count of four. As you exhale, your abdomen should move inward.

9. As the air flows out, imagine all your tension and stress leaving your body.

10. Repeat the process until you achieve a sense of deep relaxation.

THE IMPORTANCE OF SLEEP

Over the course of a year, over half of the U.S. population will have difficulty falling asleep. About 33% of the population experiences insomnia regularly. Many people use over-the-counter sedative medications to combat insomnia, while others seek stronger drugs. Insomnia can have many causes, but the most common are depression, anxiety, use of stimulants like caffeine and faulty blood sugar control. In addition, well over 300 drugs have been identified that can interfere with normal sleep.

Poor sleep quality can reduce insulin sensitivity and set the stage for increasing the risk for not only diabetes, but also CVD.

ELIMINATION OF INHIBITORS OF SLEEP

Coffee, as well as less obvious caffeine sources such as soft drinks, chocolate, coffee-flavored ice cream, hot cocoa, and tea, must all be eliminated in people who suffer from insomnia. Even small amounts of caffeine, such as those found in decaffeinated coffee or in chocolate, may be enough to cause insomnia in some people.

FIVE TIPS FOR PREPARING FOR A GOOD NIGHT'S SLEEP

1. **MAKE YOUR BEDROOM PRIMARILY A PLACE FOR SLEEPING.** It is not a good idea to use your bed for paying bills, doing work, etc. Help your body recognize that this is a place for rest or intimacy. Make sure your room is well ventilated and the temperature consistent. And try to keep it quiet. You could use a fan or a "white noise" machine to help block outside noises.

2. **INCORPORATE BEDTIME RITUALS.** Listening to soft music, sipping a cup of herbal tea, etc., cues your body that it's time to slow down and begin to prepare for sleep.

3. **RELAX FOR A WHILE BEFORE GOING TO BED.** Spending quiet time can make falling asleep easier. This may include meditation, relaxation and/ or breathing exercises, or taking a warm bath. Try listening to recorded relaxation or guided imagery programs.

4. **GET OUT OF BED IF YOU'RE UNABLE TO SLEEP.** Don't lie in bed awake. Go into another room and do something relaxing until you feel sleepy. Worrying about falling asleep actually keeps many people awake.

5. **DON'T DO ANYTHING STIMULATING.** Don't read anything job related or watch a stimulating TV program (commercials and news shows tend to make people alert). Don't expose yourself to bright light. The light cues your brain that it's time to wake up.

Other food compounds that can act as stimulants include some food colorings. Adverse food reactions such as food sensitivities and allergies can also cause insomnia. Although not considered a stimulant, sugar and refined carbohydrates can interfere with sleep. Eating a diet high in sugar and refined carbohydrate and eating irregularly can cause a reaction in the body that triggers the fight-or-flight part of the nervous system, causing wakefulness.

Alcohol must also be eliminated in people with regular insomnia. Alcohol causes the release of adrenaline and disrupts the production of serotonin (an important brain chemical that initiates sleep).

BLOOD SUGAR CONTROL AND SLEEP QUALITY

In people who have trouble maintaining sleep throughout the night, I have found faulty blood sugar control as an important cause. When the blood glucose level drops, it causes the release of hormones that regulate glucose levels, such as adrenaline, glucagon, cortisol, and growth hormone. These compounds stimulate the brain. They are a natural signal that it is time to eat. To reduce nighttime awakening due to blood sugar volatility, I recommend following the dietary guidelines given in Chapter 2, along with the recommendations for using PGX® given in Chapter 4.

SPECIAL DIETARY SUPPLEMENTS TO PROMOTE A GOOD NIGHT'S SLEEP

There are a number of special natural products that I have found to be extremely reliable in helping to improve sleep quality. Most often I recommend a product that I developed called Tranquil Sleep. This formula provides the combination of melatonin (3 mg), 5-HTP (30 mg), and L-theanine (200 mg) in a great-tasting chewable tablet or an enteric-coated soft gelatin capsule. These three ingredients work together to decrease the time required to get to sleep and to decrease the number of nighttime awakenings.

Here is the information on each of these components and dosage recommendations at bedtime:

- **MELATONIN** is an important hormone secreted by the pineal gland, a small gland in the center of the brain. Melatonin is one of the best aids for sleep. In several studies, supplementation with melatonin has been found helpful in inducing and maintaining sleep in both children and adults, for both people with normal sleep patterns and those suffering from insomnia. However, it appears that the sleep-promoting effects of melatonin are most apparent only if a person's melatonin levels are low. In other words, taking melatonin is not like taking a sleeping pill or even 5-HTP. It will produce a sedative effect only when melatonin levels are low. A dosage of 3 mg at bedtime is more than enough.

- **5-HYDROXYTRYPTOPHAN (5-HTP)** is converted in the brain to serotonin – an important initiator of sleep. 5-HTP has also been reported, in numerous double-blind clinical studies, to decrease the time required to get to sleep and to decrease the number of awakenings. The recommended dosage is 50–100 mg in a chewable tablet or enteric-coated capsule.

- **L-THEANINE** is an important consideration when trying to get a better night's sleep. At typical dosages, e.g., 100–200 mg, L-theanine does not act as a sedative, but it does significantly improve sleep quality. It is an excellent support agent for melatonin and 5-HTP. These ingredients exert synergistic effects to promote restful sleep. *Note:* At higher single dosages, e.g., 600 mg, L-theanine does exert sedative action.

As for herbal medicines to promote a good night's sleep, valerian *(Valeriana officinalis)* is by far the most popular. Several double-blind clinical studies have substantiated valerian's ability to improve sleep quality and relieve insomnia. In fact, it has shown effectiveness equal to prescription sleeping pills. The advantage of valerian is that it does not cause daytime sleepiness, diminished concentration, or impairment of physical performance. The dosage for standardized valerian extract (0.8% valerenic acid content) is 150–300 mg, 45 minutes before bedtime. I would reserve use of valerian until after you have given the combination of melatonin, 5-HTP, and L-theanine a try because I have found Tranquil Sleep to be much more effective.

THE IMPORTANCE OF REGULAR EXERCISE

Regular physical exercise is obviously a vital key to heart health. We all know this fact, yet fewer than 50% of Americans exercise regularly. While the immediate effect of exercise is stress on the body, with regular exercise the body adapts – it becomes stronger, functions more efficiently, and has greater endurance. These benefits are largely the result of improved cardiovascular function. Simply stated, exercise enhances the transport of oxygen and nutrients into cells. At the same time, exercise enhances the transport of carbon dioxide and waste products from the tissues of the body to the bloodstream and ultimately to the organs that eliminate them.

Physical inactivity is a major risk factor for heart disease and is also a key reason so many Americans are overweight. Exercise promotes the development of an efficient method of burning fat. Muscle tissue is the primary user of calories in the body, so the greater your muscle mass, the greater your fat-burning capacity. If you want to be healthy and achieve your ideal body weight, you must exercise.

Regular exercise also exerts a powerfully positive effect on mood. Tension, depression, feelings of inadequacy, and worries diminish greatly with regular exercise. Exercise alone has been demonstrated to have a tremendous impact on improving mood and the ability to handle stressful life situations.

If the benefits of exercise could be put in a pill, you would have the most powerful health-promoting medication available. Take a look at this long list of health benefits produced by regular exercise:

MUSCULOSKELETAL SYSTEM

- Increases muscle strength
- Increases flexibility of muscles and range of joint motion
- Produces stronger bones, ligaments, and tendons
- Prevents osteoporosis
- Lessens chance of injury
- Enhances posture, poise, and physique
- Improves balance

HEART AND BLOOD VESSELS

- Lowers resting heart rate
- Strengthens heart function
- Lowers blood pressure
- Improves oxygen delivery throughout the body
- Increases blood supply to muscles
- Enlarges the arteries to the heart
- Reduces heart disease risk
- Helps lower "bad" LDL cholesterol and triglycerides
- Raises HDL, the "good" cholesterol

BODILY PROCESSES

- Improves the way the body handles dietary fat
- Helps improve calcium deposition in bones
- Improves immune function
- Aids digestion and elimination
- Increases endurance and energy levels
- Promotes lean body mass and burns fat

MENTAL PROCESSES

- Provides a natural release for pent-up feelings
- Reduces tension and anxiety
- Improves mental outlook and self-esteem
- Helps relieve moderate depression
- Improves the ability to handle stress
- Improves mental function
- Relaxes and improves sleep

LONGEVITY

- Increases longevity

PHYSICAL FITNESS AND LONGEVITY

The better shape you're in physically, the greater your odds of enjoying a healthier and longer life. Most studies have shown that the risk of having a heart attack or stroke in an unfit individual is eight times greater than in a physically fit individual. Researchers have estimated that every hour of exercise leads to a two-hour increase in longevity. That is quite a return on investment.

The Aerobics Center Longitudinal Study involved 9,777 men aged 20–82 who had completed at least two preventive medical examinations at the Cooper Clinic in Dallas, Texas, from December 1970 through December 1989.5 All study participants achieved at least 85% of their age-predicted maximal heart rate (220 minus their age) during the treadmill tests at both exams. The average interval between the two exams was 4.9 years. Men were considered healthy if, in addition to normal resting and exercise electrocardiograms (EKGs), they had no history or evidence of heart attack, stroke, diabetes, or high blood pressure at both exams. Men were considered unhealthy if they had one or more of these conditions, even though they had normal resting and exercising EKGs. A total of 6,819 men were classified as healthy and 2,958 as unhealthy.

Even though by standard definitions all men in the study could be classified as fit, for the purpose of category analysis, they were further categorized by their level of fitness based on their exercise tolerance in a standard treadmill test. This measure is a sound objective indicator of physical fitness – test time has been shown to correlate positively with maximal oxygen uptake. The men were divided into five groups, with the first group being labeled unfit and groups 2–5 being categorized as fit. The higher the group number, the higher the level of fitness.

The highest age-adjusted death rate (all causes) was observed in men who were unfit at both exams (122.0 deaths per 10,000 man years); the lowest death rate was in men who were physically fit at both examinations (39.6 deaths per 10,000 man years). Furthermore, men who improved from unfit to fit between the first and subsequent examinations had an age-adjusted death rate of 67.7 per 10,000 man years, representing a reduction in mortality of 44% relative to men who remained unfit at both exams. Improvement in fitness was associated with lower death rates after adjusting for age, health status, and other risk factors for premature mortality. For each minute increase in maximal treadmill time between examinations, there was a corresponding 7.9% decrease in risk of mortality.

Follow-up studies have shown the same sort of findings. The most recent study, involving 40,718 healthy men, showed that physical fitness was strongly associated with lower CVD mortality, even in those with higher LDL levels, indicating that physical fitness can reduce some of the risk of high LDL levels.[6]

CREATING AN EFFECTIVE EXERCISE ROUTINE

Exercise is clearly one of the most powerful medicines available. Just imagine if all the benefits of exercise could be put in a pill. Unfortunately, it's not that easy. The time you spend exercising is a valuable investment in good health. Here are seven steps to follow to help you develop a successful exercise program:

STEP 1. REALIZE THE IMPORTANCE OF PHYSICAL EXERCISE

The first step is realizing just how important it is to get regular exercise. We cannot stress enough just how vital regular exercise is to your health. But as much as we stress this fact it means absolutely nothing unless it really sinks in and you accept it as well. You must make regular exercise a top priority in your life.

STEP 2. CONSULT YOUR PHYSICIAN

If you are not currently on a regular exercise program, get medical clearance if you have health problems or if you are over 40 years of age. The main concern is the functioning of your heart. Exercise can be quite harmful (and even fatal) if your heart is not able to meet the increased demands placed on it. It is especially important to see a physician if any of the following apply to you:

- Heart disease
- Smoking
- High blood pressure
- Extreme breathlessness with physical exertion
- Pain or pressure in chest, arm, teeth, jaw, or neck with exercise
- Dizziness or fainting
- Abnormal heart action (palpitations or irregular beat)

STEP 3. SELECT AN ACTIVITY YOU CAN ENJOY

If you are fit enough to begin, the next thing to do is select an activity you feel you would enjoy. From the suggestions in the next paragraph, choose one or two of the activities – or fill in a choice or two of your own – that you think you may enjoy. Make a commitment to do one activity a day for at least 20 minutes and preferably an hour. Make the enjoyment of the activity your goal. The important thing is to move your body enough to raise your pulse a bit above its resting rate.

The best exercises for your heart are those that elevate your heart rate the most. Aerobic activities such as walking briskly, jogging, bicycling, cross-country skiing, swimming, aerobic dance, and racquet sports are good examples. Brisk walking (five miles an hour) for approximately 30 minutes may be the very best form of exercise for weight loss. Walking can be done anywhere; it doesn't require any expensive equipment, just comfortable clothing and well-fitting shoes, and the risk for injury is extremely low. If you are going to walk regularly, we strongly urge you to first purchase a pair of high-quality walking or jogging shoes.

STEP 4. MONITOR EXERCISE INTENSITY

Exercise intensity is determined by measuring your heart rate (the number of times your heart beats per minute). You can determine this quickly by placing the index and middle fingers of one hand on the side of your neck just below the angle of the jaw or on the inside of the opposite wrist. Beginning with zero, count the number of heartbeats for six seconds. Simply add a zero to this number and you have your pulse. For example, if you counted 14 beats, your heart rate would be 140. Would this be a good number? It depends on your "training zone."

A quick and easy way to determine your maximum training heart rate is to simply subtract your age from 185. For example, if you are 40 your maximum heart rate is 145. To determine the bottom of the training zone, simply subtract 20 from this number. In the case of a 40-year-old this would be 125; the training range would be a heartbeat of 125–145 beats per minute. For maximum health benefits you must stay in this range but never exceed it.

STEP 5. DO IT OFTEN

You don't get in good physical condition by exercising once; you must exercise regularly. A minimum of 15–20 minutes of exercise at your training heart rate at least three times a week is necessary to gain any significant cardiovascular benefits from exercise.

STEP 6. MAKE IT FUN

The key to getting the maximum benefit from exercise is to make it enjoyable. Choose an activity you enjoy and have fun doing. If you can find enjoyment in exercise, you are much more likely to exercise regularly. One way to make it fun is to get a workout partner. For example, if you choose walking as your activity, here's a great way to make it fun: Find one or two people in your neighborhood with whom you would enjoy walking. If you are meeting one or two people, you will certainly walk more regularly than if you depend solely on your own intentions. Commit to walking 3–5 mornings or afternoons each week, and increase the exercise duration from an initial 10 minutes to at least 30 minutes.

STEP 7. STAY MOTIVATED

No matter how committed a person is to regular exercise, at some point they are going to be faced with a loss of enthusiasm for working out. Here is a suggestion: take a break. Not a long break, just skip one or two workouts. It gives your enthusiasm and motivation a chance to recoup so you can come back with an even stronger commitment. Here are some other strategies to help you to stay motivated:

- **SET EXERCISE GOALS.** Being goal oriented helps keep us motivated. Success breeds success, so set a lot of small goals you can easily achieve. Write down your daily exercise goal and check it off when you have completed it.

- **VARY YOUR ROUTINE.** Variety is very important to help you stay interested in exercise. Doing the same thing every day becomes monotonous and drains motivation. Continually find new ways to enjoy working out.

- **KEEP A RECORD OF YOUR ACTIVITIES AND PROGRESS.** Sometimes it's hard to see the progress you're making, but if you write in a journal you'll have a permanent record of your progress. Keeping track of your progress will motivate you to continued improvement.

FINAL COMMENTS

The importance of a health-promoting lifestyle cannot be overstated. Lifestyle definitely comes down to choices. If you want to be healthy, simply make healthy choices. Choose not to smoke. Choose to find physical activities you enjoy and do them often. Make getting a good night's sleep a priority. Take time out to relax and "sharpen the saw." What do I mean by that? In the book *The 7 Habits of Highly Effective People*, author Stephen R. Covey made famous the following analogy:

Suppose you were to come upon someone in the woods working feverishly to saw down a tree.

"What are you doing?" you ask.

"Can't you see?" comes the impatient reply. *"I'm sawing down this tree."*

"You look exhausted!" you exclaim. *"How long have you been at it?"*

"Over five hours," he returns, *"and I'm beat! This is hard work."*

"Well, why don't you take a break for a few minutes and sharpen that saw?" you inquire. *"I'm sure it would go a lot faster."*

"I don't have time to sharpen the saw," the man says emphatically. *"I'm too busy sawing!"*

For me, sharpening the saw is working out, scheduling a nap or time for relaxation exercises, and, of course, spending time with my family. If you want a full life, you have got to schedule those types of activities – they will keep your saw sharp. Every night I plan out the following day by creating a prioritized to-do list and then schedule my day in 15-minute increments. I always plan some flex time to catch up or sharpen the saw. It helps me keep my type A behavior in check and reminds me what is really important.

CHAPTER 6

HIGH BLOOD PRESSURE

High blood pressure, or hypertension, is a major risk factor for a heart attack or stroke. In fact, it is generally regarded as the most significant risk factor for a stroke. More than 60 million Americans have high blood pressure, including more than half (54.3%) of all Americans age 65–74 years and almost three quarters (71.8%) of all African Americans in the same age group.

High blood pressure is most often due to atherosclerosis (hardening of the arteries). As a result, it leads to disruption of the regulation of the degree of constriction of blood vessels and fluid volume. Although genetic factors play a role, there is little debate that dietary, lifestyle, psychological, and environmental factors are the underlying causes in most cases of high blood pressure. Some of the important lifestyle factors include smoking, stress, and lack of exercise. The most important dietary factors are obesity; high sodium to potassium ratio; a low-fiber, high-sugar diet; high saturated fat and low essential omega-3 fatty acid intake; and a diet low in magnesium. These dietary and lifestyle factors were discussed in Chapters 2 and 5. In addition, since being overweight and having insulin resistance are major factors in so many people with high blood pressure, the recommendations in Chapter 4 are important, especially the use of PGX®.

Table 6.1 Classification of Blood Pressure

OPTIMAL
- Systolic below 120 mm Hg
- Diastolic below 80 mm Hg

NORMAL
- Systolic below 130 mm Hg
- Diastolic below 85 mm Hg

BORDERLINE (HIGH-NORMAL)
- Systolic 130–139 mm Hg
- Diastolic 85–89 mm Hg

HIGH BLOOD PRESSURE
- Stage 1 (mild):
  - Systolic 140–159 mm Hg
  - Diastolic 90–99 mm Hg
- Stage 2 (moderate):
  - Systolic 160–179 mm Hg
  - Diastolic 100–109 mm Hg
- Stage 3 (severe):
  - Systolic 180 mm Hg or above
  - Diastolic 110 mm Hg or above

ADVANTAGES OF NATURAL APPROACHES TO LOWERING BLOOD PRESSURE

Because more than 80% of patients with high blood pressure are in the borderline to moderate range, most cases of high blood pressure can be brought under control through changes in diet and lifestyle. Therefore, it can be concluded that up to 80% of the prescriptions for high blood pressure are ill advised. In fact, in head-to-head comparisons, many nondrug therapies such as diet, exercise, and relaxation therapies have proved to be superior to drugs in cases of borderline to mild hypertension.

And, here is another important point: several well-designed, long-term clinical studies have found that people taking diuretics or beta blockers – or both – actually suffered not only from unnecessary side effects, but also showed an increased risk for heart disease and diabetes. Now keep in mind that the reason high blood pressure is treated is to reduce the risk for heart disease and strokes. Although the newer class of drugs, the calcium channel blockers and angiotensin-converting enzyme (ACE) inhibitors, appear to be safer and have fewer side effects, they are also not without problems – nearly every patient taking these drugs experiences some sort of side effect. Most are mild, but annoying nonetheless.

ANTIHYPERTENSIVE DRUGS

The four major categories of blood pressure lowering drugs are diuretics, beta blockers, calcium channel blockers, and ACE inhibitors. Here is a brief description of each drug, followed by current recommendations for the drug treatment of high blood pressure.

DIURETICS

Diuretics lower blood pressure by reducing the volume of fluid in the blood and body tissues by promoting the elimination of salt and water through increased urination. In addition, diuretics also work to relax the smaller arteries of the body, allowing them to expand and increase the total fluid capacity of the arterial system. The net result of diuretics is lower pressure due to reduced volume in an expanded space. By far the most popular type are thiazide diuretics; they are often the first drug used in treating mild to moderate high blood pressure.

The following are examples of thiazide diuretics:

- Bendroflumethiazide (Naturetin)

- Benzthiazide (Exna, Hydrex)

- Chlorothiazide (Diuril), chlorthalidone (Hydone, Hygroton, Novo-Thalidone, Thalitone, Uridon), and cyclothiazide (Anhydron)

- Hydrochlorothiazide (Apo-Hydro, Diuchlor H, Esidrix, Hydro-chlor, HydroDIURIL, Neo-Codema, Novo-Hydrazide, Oretic, Urozide)

- Hydroflumethiazide (Diucardin, Saluron)

- Methyclothiazide (Aquatensen, Duretic, Enduron)

- Metolazone (Diulo, Mykrox, Zaroxolyn)

- Polythiazide (Renese)

- Quinethazone (Hydromox)

- Trichlormethiazide (Aquazide, Diurese, Metahydrin, Naqua, Trichlorex)

Some of the side effects of thiazide diuretics are light-headedness, increased blood sugar levels, increased uric acid levels, aggravation of gout, and muscle weakness and cramps caused by low potassium levels. Decreased libido and impotence are also reported. Less-frequent side effects include allergic reactions, headaches, blurred vision, nausea, vomiting, and diarrhea.

Thiazide diuretics also cause the loss of potassium, magnesium, and calcium from the body. These minerals have all been shown to exert blood pressure lowering effects and prevent heart attacks. The drugs also increase cholesterol and triglyceride levels; increase the viscosity of the blood; raise uric acid levels; and increase the stickiness of the platelets, making them likely to aggregate and form clots. All of these factors may explain why thiazide diuretics may actually increase the risk of dying from a heart attack or stroke. Thiazide diuretics also have a tendency to worsen blood sugar control, making them difficult to use safely in diabetics.

BETA BLOCKERS

Beta blockers reduce the rate and force of the contraction of the heart and relax the arteries. In addition to high blood pressure, beta blockers are also used in treating angina and certain heart rhythm disturbances. Because heart function is reduced with beta blockers, there is a decreased need for oxygen and angina is relieved. In the long term, however, this inhibition of heart function can lead to heart failure. Beta blockers have fallen out of favor owing to the lack of effectiveness in reducing cardiovascular mortality and because they have been shown to increase the risk of developing diabetes by about 30%.

Beta blockers produce some significant side effects in many patients. Because cardiac output is reduced in a more relaxed arterial system, it is often difficult to get enough blood and oxygen to the hands, feet, and brain. This results in the typical symptoms described by users of beta blockers, such as cold hands and feet, nerve tingling, impaired mental function, fatigue, dizziness, depression, lethargy, reduced libido, and impotence. Beta blockers also raise cholesterol and triglyceride levels considerably. This may explain some of the negative effects in the clinical studies, which failed to demonstrate any significant benefit of beta blockers in reducing mortality from cardiovascular disease.

It is extremely important that a beta blocker not be discontinued suddenly. Stopping the medication suddenly can produce a withdrawal syndrome consisting of headache, increased heart rate, and dramatic increase in blood pressure.

The following are examples of beta blockers:

- Acebutolol (Sectral, Prent)
- Atenolol (Senormin, Tenormin)
- Bisoprolol fumarate (Zebeta)
- Carteolol (Cartrol, Ocupress)
- Metoprolol succinate (Toprol-XL)
- Metoprolol tartrate (Lopressor)
- Nadolol (Corgard)
- Penbutolol sulfate (Levatol)
- Pindolol (Visken)
- Propranolol (Betachron, Inderal, Pronol)
- Timolol maleate (Blocadren, Timoptic)

CALCIUM CHANNEL BLOCKERS

Calcium channel blocking drugs, along with ACE inhibitors, have taken over the top spots in the drug treatment of high blood pressure because they are better tolerated than diuretics and beta blockers. Although calcium channel blockers have been shown to lower the risk of stroke, they carry the same increased risk for heart attacks as the older approach of diuretics and beta blockers.

Calcium channel blockers work by blocking the normal passage of calcium through certain channels in cell walls. Since calcium is required in the function of nerve transmission and muscle contraction, the effect of blocking the calcium channel is to slow down nerve conduction and inhibit the contraction of the muscle. In the heart and vascular system, this action results in reducing the rate and force of contraction, relaxing the arteries, and slowing the nerve impulses in the heart.

Although much better tolerated than beta blockers and diuretics, calcium channel blockers still produce some mild side effects, including constipation, allergic reactions, fluid retention, dizziness, headache, fatigue, and impotence (in about 20% of users). More serious side effects include disturbances of heart rate or function, heart failure, and angina.

The following are examples of calcium channel blockers:

- Amlodipine (Norvasc)
- Diltiazem (Cardizem CD, Cartia XT, Dilacor XR, Diltia XT, Tiazac)
- Felodipine (Plendil)
- Lacidipine (Motens)
- Lercanidipine (Zanidip)
- Nicardipine (Cardene, Cardene SR)
- Nifedipine (Adalat CC, Procardia XL)
- Nimodipine (Nimotop)
- Nisoldipine (Sular)
- Nitrendipine (Cardif, Nitrepin)
- Verapamil (Calan, Covera-HS, Isoptin, Verelan)

ANGIOTENSIN-CONVERTING ENZYME INHIBITORS

ACE inhibitors prevent the formation of angiotensin II, a substance that increases both the fluid volume and the degree of constriction of the blood vessels. ACE inhibitors relax the arterial walls and reduce fluid volume. Unlike the beta blockers and calcium channel blockers, however, ACE inhibitors actually improve heart function and increase blood and oxygen flow to the heart, liver, and kidneys. This effect may explain why ACE inhibitors are the only blood pressure drugs that appear to reduce the risk of heart attacks. Unfortunately, they do not have any effect on reducing the risk for strokes.

The newer ACE inhibitors are generally well tolerated but share many of the same side effects as other blood pressure medications, including dizziness, light-headedness, and headache. The most common side effect is a dry nighttime cough. ACE inhibitors can also cause potassium buildup and kidney problems, so potassium levels and kidney function must be monitored.

The following are examples of ACE inhibitors:

- Benazepril (Lotensin)
- Captopril (Capoten)
- Captopril/hydrochlorothiazide (Capozide)
- Enalapril maleate (Vasotec, Renitec)
- Fosinopril sodium (Monopril)
- Lisinopril (Lisodur, Lopril, Novatec, Prinivil, Zestril)
- Perindopril (Coversyl, Aceon)
- Quinapril/magnesium carbonate (Accupril)
- Ramipril (Altace, Tritace, Ramace, Ramiwin)
- Trandolapril (Mavik)

CURRENT DRUG TREATMENT OF HIGH BLOOD PRESSURE

For many years the drug of first choice for high blood pressure was a thiazide diuretic alone or in combination with a beta blocker. As mentioned earlier, because of the lack of effectiveness in reducing the cardiovascular death rate, and because of the side effects noted in numerous studies, this approach has somewhat fallen out of favor. Currently, the most commonly used medication is a diuretic used alone or in combination with newer medications designed to relax the arteries, such as calcium channel blockers and ACE inhibitors.

The use of a diuretic or any of these other drugs alone is referred to as a step 1 approach. Thiazide diuretics are still the most popular step 1 drug but may soon be displaced by calcium channel blockers or ACE inhibitors. Beta blockers are not suitable as step 1 drugs owing to their known side effects. A step 2 drug approach uses two medications, a step 3 approach uses three, and a step 4 approach is composed of four medications. Physicians are instructed to use single therapies before combinations of medicines. Of course, they are also instructed to use nondrug therapies first, but that rarely occurs.

HIGH BLOOD PRESSURE – A RATIONAL APPROACH

There is no question that in most cases of high blood pressure, nondrug therapy is more than effective at bringing the numbers down into the normal range. For moderate through severe hypertension, drug therapy may be necessary initially until the dietary, lifestyle, and supplement strategies take hold. However, sometimes long-term drug therapy is required, especially in moderate to severe hypertension, but that does not mean that dietary and lifestyle strategies should be abandoned.

KEY DIETARY RECOMMENDATIONS

The most important long-term dietary goal for most patients with high blood pressure is achieving normal body weight. Obesity is the major dietary cause of high blood pressure. From borderline high blood pressure all the way to chronic renal failure, weight loss can lead to complete elimination of the health issue, significant improvement, or at least reduction in the number of prescription drugs a person is taking.[1,2]

Next to attaining ideal body weight, another very important dietary recommendation is to eat a low-sodium, high-potassium diet. Between 40% and 60% of people with high blood pressure are salt sensitive. That means that following a sodium-restricted diet will normalize their blood pressure. Despite this fact, most doctors do not prescribe a low-sodium, high-potassium diet because they view it as being "inconvenient." But it is not as inconvenient as a stroke or the side effects of the drugs often prescribed to treat high blood pressure. A salt-restricted diet simply makes great practical sense and may be entirely curative.

It is also important to increase the proportion of plant foods in the diet. Vegetarians generally have lower blood pressure levels and a lower incidence of high blood pressure and other cardiovascular diseases than nonvegetarians.[3] Although dietary levels of sodium do not differ significantly between these two groups, a vegetarian's diet typically contains more potassium, complex carbohydrates, beneficial oils, fiber, calcium, magnesium, and vitamin C and less saturated fat and refined carbohydrates, all of which have a favorable influence on blood pressure.

Increasing fruit and vegetable intake has been shown to lower blood pressure.[4] This effect may be the result of increasing antioxidant concentrations. People with high blood pressure have been shown to have increased oxidative stress and dietary antioxidants have been shown to produce some benefits in high blood pressure.[5,6]

The most useful foods for people with high blood pressure include the following:

- Celery
- Garlic and onions
- Nuts and seeds or their oils for their essential fatty acid content
- Cold-water fish (e.g., salmon, mackerel)
- Green leafy vegetables for their calcium and magnesium
- Whole grains and legumes for their fiber
- Foods rich in vitamin C, such as broccoli and citrus fruits
- Foods rich in active flavonoids, including berries, cherries, grapes, and small red kidney beans

Celery is a particularly interesting recommendation for high blood pressure. It contains 3-n-butylphthalide (3nB), a compound that has been found to lower blood pressure. In animals, a small amount of this compound lowered blood pressure by 12–14% and cholesterol by about 7%.[7] The equivalent dose in humans can be supplied in about 4–6 ribs of celery. The research was prompted by the father of one of the researchers, who, after eating a quarter pound of celery daily for one week, observed that his blood pressure had dropped from 158/96 to 118/82 mm Hg. Celery seed extract can also lower blood pressure. Take an extract providing 85% 3nB at a dosage of 75–150 mg twice daily.

Garlic and onions are also important foods for lowering blood pressure. Although most recent research has focused on the cholesterol-lowering properties of garlic and onions, both have also been shown to lower high blood pressure. Commercial garlic supplements may also be of benefit.

A detailed analysis of published clinical trials of garlic preparations was conducted to determine the effect of garlic on blood pressure relative to placebo.[8] Eight trials (seven double blind, one single blind) were identified as meeting analytic criteria. A total of 415 people were included in the analysis. All trials used a dried garlic powder standardized to contain 1.3% alliin at a dosage of 600–900 mg daily (corresponding to 7.8–11.7 mg of alliin, or the equivalent of approximately 1.8–2.7 g of fresh garlic daily). The analysis concluded that garlic preparations designed to yield allicin can lower systolic and diastolic blood pressures over a 1–3 month period. The typical drop from pooled data was 11 mm Hg in systolic pressure and 5 mm Hg in diastolic pressure.

THE DIETARY APPROACHES TO STOP HYPERTENSION DIET

The Dietary Approaches to Stop Hypertension (DASH) clinical studies were funded by the National Heart, Lung, and Blood Institute to fully evaluate the efficacy of a system of dietary recommendations in the treatment of high blood pressure. The DASH diet is rich in fruit, vegetables, and low-fat dairy foods and low in saturated and total fat. It is also low in cholesterol; high in dietary fiber, potassium, calcium, and magnesium; and moderately high in protein.

The first study showed that a diet rich in fruit, vegetables, and low-fat dairy products can reduce blood pressure in the general population and in people with high blood pressure.[9] The original DASH diet did not require either sodium restriction or weight loss – the two traditional dietary tools to control blood pressure – to be effective.[10] The second study from the DASH research group found that coupling the original DASH diet with sodium restriction is more effective than either dietary change alone.[11]

In the first trial, the DASH diet produced a net blood pressure reduction of 11.4 and 5.5 mm Hg in systolic and diastolic pressure, respectively, in patients with high blood pressure. In the second trial, sodium intake was also quantified at a "higher" intake of 3300 mg/day, an "intermediate" intake of 2400 mg/day, and a "lower" intake of 1500 mg/day. Compared with the control diet, the DASH diet was associated with a significantly lower systolic blood pressure at each sodium level. The DASH diet with the lower sodium level led to an average systolic blood pressure that was 7.1 mm Hg lower in participants without high blood pressure and 11.5 mm Hg lower in those with the condition.

These results are clinically significant and indicate that a sodium intake below 1500 mg daily can significantly and quickly lower blood pressure. Table 6.2 provides a brief description of the components of the DASH eating plan on the basis of a 2000-calorie daily diet.

Table 6.2 Components of the DASH Eating Plan (2000-calorie daily diet)

Food Group	Daily Servings	Serving Sizes	Examples	Significance of each Food Group to the DASH Diet Pattern
Vegetables	4–5	1 cup raw leafy vegetable ½ cup cooked vegetable 6 oz vegetable juice	Artichokes, beans, broccoli, carrots, collards, kale, peas, potatoes, spinach, squash, sweet potatoes, tomatoes, turnip greens	Rich sources of potassium, magnesium, and fiber

Food Group	Daily Servings	Serving Sizes	Examples	Significance of each Food Group to the DASH Diet Pattern
Fruit	4–5	6 oz fruit juice 1 medium fruit ¼ cup dried fruit ½ cup fresh, frozen, or canned fruit	Apricots, bananas, dates, grapefruit, grapefruit juice, mangoes, melons, oranges, orange juice, peaches, pineapples, prunes, raisins, strawberries, tangerines	Important sources of potassium, magnesium, and fiber
Low-fat or nonfat dairy foods	2–3	8 oz milk 1 cup yogurt 1.5 oz cheese	Skim or 1% milk, skim or low-fat buttermilk, nonfat or low-fat yogurt, part skim mozzarella cheese, nonfat cheese	Major sources of calcium and protein
Meat, poultry, and fish	2 or fewer	3 oz cooked meat, poultry, or fish	Select only lean meat; trim away visible fat; remove skin from poultry; broil, roast, or boil instead of frying	Rich sources of protein and magnesium
Nuts, seeds, and legumes	4–5 per week	1½ oz or ⅓ cup nuts ½ oz or 2 tbsp seeds ½ cup cooked legumes	Almonds, filberts, mixed nuts, peanuts, walnuts, sunflower seeds, kidney beans, lentils	Rich sources of energy, magnesium, potassium, protein, and fiber

ANTI-ACE PEPTIDES

Various naturally occurring peptides have been shown to inhibit the angiotensin-converting enzyme (ACE) that leads to the formation of a compound (angiotensin II) that causes large blood vessels to constrict and the kidneys to hold on to more sodium. The most studied of these peptides is composed of a purified mixture of nine small peptides (proteins) derived from muscle of the fish bonito (a member of the tuna family).[12–15] Anti-ACE bonito peptides do not appear to produce the side effects typical of ACE inhibitor drugs according to human safety studies and do not lower blood pressure in people with normal blood pressure, even when administered at levels 20 times greater than the dosage that lowers blood pressure in people with high blood pressure. A possible reason is that the mechanism of action of bonito peptides in inhibiting ACEs is different from that of the drugs.

Research bears out this theory. The drugs basically indiscriminately block ACEs by interfering with their action, while the bonito anti-ACE peptides interact much differently. ACEs convert angiotensin I to angiotensin II by cleaving off a small peptide. Drugs work by directly blocking this action. Naturally occurring anti-ACE peptides work differently, as ACEs actually react with the peptides instead of angiotensin. In addition to competing with angiotensin through this effect, anti-ACE peptides are transformed into even more potent inhibitors of ACEs. Technically, the bonito anti-ACE peptides are considered a "pro-drug" because the transformed peptides exert 800% greater activity.

Four clinical studies have shown that fish-derived anti-ACE peptides (three with the bonito peptides and one with a dipeptide from sardine) exert significant blood pressure lowering effects in people with high blood pressure.[13–16] The degree of blood pressure reduction in these studies was quite significant, typically reducing the systolic pressure by at least 10 mm Hg and the diastolic pressure by 7 mm Hg in people with borderline and mild hypertension. Greater reductions are seen in people with higher initial blood pressure readings.

COENZYME Q$_{10}$

Coenzyme Q$_{10}$ (CoQ$_{10}$), also known as ubiquinone, is an essential component of the mitochondria. Although the body can make CoQ$_{10}$, deficiencies have been reported, especially in people taking statin drugs. In high blood pressure, CoQ$_{10}$ deficiency has been shown to be present in 39% of patients. This finding alone suggests a need for CoQ$_{10}$ supplementation. However, CoQ$_{10}$ appears to provide benefits beyond correction of a deficiency.

A detailed review on CoQ$_{10}$ in the treatment of high blood pressure (12 clinical trials, 362 patients) concluded that in hypertensive patients, CoQ$_{10}$ has the potential to lower systolic and diastolic blood pressure, without significant side effects.[17] Among all included studies, decreases in systolic blood pressure ranged from 11 to 17 mm Hg and in diastolic pressure from 8 to 10 mm Hg. In three of the 12 studies, CoQ10 was given in addition to existing blood pressure medication, and in one of these more than 50% of the patients were able to cease taking at least one medication during the trial.

These results are consistent with some of the uncontrolled studies. For example, in one uncontrolled study, the dosage of CoQ10 was adjusted in 109 patients with high blood pressure according to clinical response and blood CoQ10 levels (the aim was to attain blood levels above 2 mcg/ml). The average CoQ10 dose was 225 mg/day in addition to their usual blood pressure medications. The need for medications declined gradually, and after an average treatment period of 4.4 months, about half the patients were able to discontinue 1–3 of their drugs.[18]

It is important to keep in mind that the blood pressure lowering effect of CoQ10 is usually not seen until after 4–12 weeks of therapy. Thus CoQ10 is not a typical blood pressure lowering drug; rather, it seems to correct some metabolic abnormality, which in turn has a favorable influence on blood pressure.

BOTANICAL MEDICINES THAT LOWER HYPERTENSION

OLIVE *(OLEA EUROPAEA)*

The leaves of the olive tree *(Olea europaea L.)* have been used since ancient times to combat high blood pressure and have received significant support in recent animal and human studies both for high blood pressure and for lowering cholesterol. The active substances are oleuropein (a polyphenolic iridoid glycoside),[19] oleacein, and oleanolic acid, which act as natural calcium channel blocking agents to relax constricted large blood vessels. Hydroxytyrosol is a metabolite of oleuropein that exerts antioxidant effects. Often olive extracts are standardized for hydroxytyrosol, but this compound is devoid of any significant effect on blood pressure. Oleuropein is also found in the fruit and oil, but in significantly smaller quantities than in the leaf.

In an initial small, double-blind study of patients with high blood pressure, 12 consulting a doctor for the first time and 18 currently on blood pressure drugs, olive leaf extract at a dosage of 400 mg four times daily for three months produced a modest yet statistically significant decrease in blood pressure with no side effects.[20]

More recent studies have used an extract standardized to oleuropein (16–24%) and polyphenols. In a preliminary clinical study carried out in 20 adult identical twins with mild hypertension, one of the twins in each pair received either a dose of 500 or 1000 mg daily and the other twin took a matching placebo. After eight weeks, systolic blood pressure remained unchanged from baseline in the placebo group and the 500 mg/ day group, but had significantly decreased for the 1000 mg/day group (137 vs. 126 mm Hg).[21]

In another study, 232 patients with high blood pressure were given either the olive leaf extract (500 mg twice daily) or the conventional antihypertensive drug captopril (12.5 mg twice daily). Average blood pressure at baseline was 149.3/93.9 mm Hg in the olive group and 148.4/93.8 mm Hg in the captopril group. Averages of systolic blood pressure reduction from baseline to the end of study were 11.5 and 13.7 mm Hg in the olive and captopril groups, respectively; diastolic pressure was reduced 4.8 and 6.4 mm Hg, respectively.[22]

HIBISCUS SABDARIFFA

Hibiscus tea and extracts prepared from the dried flowers (calyces) of *Hibiscus sabdariffa* have demonstrated blood pressure lowering properties in clinical trials. The active components are anthocyanidin glycosides. One double-blind trial was conducted in 65 adults aged 30–70 years with borderline or mildly high blood pressure not taking blood pressure medications. They received either three 240 ml servings per day of brewed hibiscus tea or a placebo beverage for six weeks. At six weeks, hibiscus tea had lowered systolic blood pressure more than placebo had (a reduction of 7.2 vs. 1.3 mm Hg). Diastolic pressure was also lower, although this change did not differ from the change with placebo. Participants with higher systolic pressure at baseline showed a greater response to hibiscus treatment.[23]

In another double-blind study, the effect of hibiscus tea was compared with that of black tea in 60 diabetic patients with mild hypertension, but not taking blood pressure or lipid-lowering drugs. The average systolic blood pressure in the hibiscus group decreased from 134.4 mm Hg at the beginning of the study to 112.7 mm Hg after one month, while it increased from 118.6 to 127.3 mm Hg in the black tea group. The interventions had no statistically significant effect on the average diastolic blood pressure in either group.[24]

Another study with hibiscus tea did show an effect on diastolic blood pressure (reduced by 10.7%) as well as systolic pressure (reduced by 11.2%) after 12 days of treatment.[25]

Two clinical studies featured a standardized extract of hibiscus. In one double-blind study, 193 patients with high blood pressure were given either hibiscus extract (250 mg of total anthocyanins daily) or 10 mg of lisinopril (control group). Results showed that the hibiscus extract decreased blood pressure from 146.48/97.77 to 129.89/85.96 mm Hg, reaching an absolute reduction of 17.14/11.97 mm Hg. The hibiscus treatment showed therapeutic effectiveness of 65.12% as well as tolerability and safety of 100%. Blood pressure reductions and therapeutic effectiveness were lower than those obtained with lisinopril. Hibiscus treatment lowered plasma ACE activity from 44.049 to 30.1 Units.[26]

Similar results on blood pressure were shown in another double-blind study with a standardized hibiscus extract (daily dosage of 9.6 mg of total anthocyanins), comparing it with another drug (captopril 50 mg/day). Results showed no significant differences in lowering blood pressure between the two treatments. Hibiscus extract was able to decrease the systolic blood pressure from 139.05 to 123.73 mm Hg and the diastolic pressure from 90.81 to 79.52 mm Hg.[27]

FINAL COMMENTS

A comprehensive program is recommended that uses lifestyle, dietary, and supplemental strategies to lower blood pressure. Again, the key goal in most people with high blood pressure is to achieve ideal body weight. Here are my concise recommendations for the various forms of high blood pressure.

BORDERLINE (130-139/85-89) OR MILD (140-159/90-99) HYPERTENSION

- Achieve ideal body weight.

- Substantially decrease salt (sodium chloride) intake.

- Follow a heart healthy lifestyle. Avoid alcohol, caffeine, and smoking. Exercise and use stress-reduction techniques.

- Follow a high-potassium diet rich in fiber and consistent with either the Mediterranean or DASH Diet and the dietary recommendations given in Chapter 2.

- Increase dietary consumption of celery, garlic, and onions.

- Reduce or eliminate the intake of animal fats while increasing the intake of monounsaturated vegetable oils.

- Supplement the diet with the following:

  · High-potency multivitamin and mineral formula

  · Vitamin C: 500–1000 mg three times daily

  · Magnesium (preferably citrate): 150–250 mg 2–3 times daily

  · Garlic: equivalent of 4000 mg of fresh garlic daily

  · Fish oils: 3000 mg total EPA+DHA content daily

If after following these recommendations for three months blood pressure has not returned to normal, follow the recommendations below.

MODERATE HYPERTENSION (160–179/100–109)

Employ all the measures listed above and add the following:

- Nattokinase: 100 mg (2000 FU) twice daily
- CoQ$_{10}$: 200–300 mg daily
- Anti-ACE peptides from bonito: 1500 mg daily
- Take one of the following:
    - Celery seed extract (85% n-butylphthalide): 75–150 mg twice daily
    - Hawthorn extract (10% procyanidins or 1.8% vitexin-4'-rhamnoside): 100–250 mg three times daily
    - Olive leaf extract (17–23% oleuropein content): 500 mg twice daily
    - Hibiscus: three 240 ml servings of hibiscus tea daily or an extract providing 10–20 mg anthocyanidins daily

These guidelines should be followed for 1–3 months. If blood pressure has not dropped below 140/105 mm Hg, medications may be required.

SEVERE HYPERTENSION (180/110 OR HIGHER)

Drug intervention is required. All the measures mentioned above should be employed as well. When satisfactory control of high blood pressure has been achieved, it may be possible to taper off the medication gradually under a physician's supervision.

CHAPTER 7

IMPROVING HEART FUNCTION, PLUS SOME SPECIAL CONSIDERATIONS
(ANGIOGRAMS, BYPASS, CHELATION, AND STROKE RECOVERY)

Whether the issue is angina, arrhythmia, cardiomyopathy, or congestive heart failure (CHF), from a naturopathic perspective the goals are very similar: improve the blood flow to the heart muscle and the functional capacity of the heart. In some cases the natural approach to these conditions will provide all the support the heart needs to function effectively. However, many of these heart conditions can be quite serious, requiring careful treatment with prescription medications and close monitoring.

We will look at some natural approaches to improving heart function as well as some special considerations, such as the use of natural products in people taking blood thinners, and when angioplasty and bypass surgeries are advised and when they are not. We will also examine intravenous ethylenediaminetetraacetic acid (EDTA) chelation therapy.

IMPROVING HEART FUNCTION

Improving energy production within the heart muscle (myocardium) is an important goal in any heart condition. Whether the issue is angina, arrhythmia, or heart failure, heart conditions are always characterized by impaired energy production within the myocardium. This impaired energy production is often the result of nutrient or coenzyme deficiency (e.g., magnesium, thiamin, coenzyme Q_{10} [CoQ_{10}], carnitine, pantethine). The dietary recommendations given in Chapters 2, 4, and 6 are definitely important. In addition, the basic supplementation strategy is also critical – a high-potency multiple, fish oils, and grape seed or pine bark extract.

MAGNESIUM

A low magnesium level (particularly in white blood cells) is a common finding in patients with angina, arrhythmia, or CHF. This association is extremely significant because magnesium levels have been shown to correlate directly with survival rates. In addition, in the case of angina or arrhythmia, sometimes magnesium supplementation can produce immediate and permanent relief. There are many clinical studies that show magnesium supplementation to be of benefit in treating angina and many types of arrhythmias, including atrial fibrillation.[1–4]

In addition, magnesium supplementation also prevents the magnesium depletion caused by the conventional drug therapy for various heart conditions. Drugs like diuretics and vasodilators, such as beta blockers and calcium channel blockers, can cause low magnesium levels. However, magnesium supplementation is not indicated in patients with kidney failure because this condition predisposes them to elevations in magnesium (hypermagnesemia). If you are a candidate for dialysis or on dialysis, do not take magnesium supplements unless instructed to do so by your physician.

For best results, use a highly bioavailable form of magnesium, such as magnesium citrate or malate. Typical dosages are 150–250 mg 2–3 times per day.

THIAMIN

Interest has recently risen regarding the potential role of thiamin deficiency in patients on diuretics. Thiamin was the first B vitamin discovered, hence its designation as vitamin B1. It is well established that thiamin deficiency can result in the cardiovascular manifestations of "wet" beriberi, sodium retention, peripheral vasodilation, and heart failure. It is also well established that furosemide (Lasix), the most widely prescribed diuretic, can cause thiamin deficiency in animals and patients with CHF.

The association between thiamin deficiency and long-term furosemide use was discovered in 1980, when it was shown that after only four weeks of furosemide use, thiamin concentrations and the activity of the thiamin-dependent enzyme transketolase were significantly reduced. The first study looking at thiamin as a potential support aid in the treatment of CHF showed only modest benefits. However, several subsequent studies have shown that daily doses of 80–240 mg of thiamin improved the clinical picture, as measured by a 13–22% increase in the left ventricular ejection fraction, a marker that tells us that thiamin improved the heart's ability to perform.[5,6] This increase is quite significant – an increase in ejection fraction is associated with a greater survival rate in patients with CHF. One study found biochemical evidence of severe thiamin deficiency in 98% of patients receiving at least 80 mg/day of furosemide and in 57% of patients taking 40 mg/day.[7]

Given the possible benefit, lack of risk, and low cost of thiamin supplementation, administration of 200–250 mg of thiamin daily appears to be a wise recommendation in patients with CHF, especially if they are on a diuretic like furosemide.

CARNITINE

Carnitine, a vitamin-like compound, stimulates the breakdown of long-chain fatty acids by the energy-producing units in cells – the mitochondria. Carnitine is essential in the transport of fatty acids into the mitochondria. A deficiency in carnitine results in a decrease in fatty acid concentrations in the mitochondria and reduced energy production.

Normal heart function is critically dependent on adequate concentrations of carnitine. Although the normal heart stores more carnitine than it needs, if the heart does not have a good supply of oxygen, carnitine levels become depleted. This leads to decreased energy production in the heart and increased risk for angina and heart disease. Since angina patients have a decreased supply of oxygen, carnitine supplementation makes good sense.

Several clinical trials have demonstrated that carnitine improves angina and heart disease. Supplementation with carnitine normalizes heart carnitine levels and allows the heart muscle to use its limited oxygen supply more efficiently. Improvements have been noted in exercise tolerance and heart function. The results indicate that carnitine is an effective alternative to drugs in many cases.

In one study of patients with stable angina, oral administration of 900 mg of carnitine increased average exercise time and the time before abnormalities occurred on a stress test (6.4 minutes in the placebo group, compared with 8.8 minutes in the carnitine-treated group).[8] These results indicate that carnitine may be an effective alternative to other anti-anginal agents such as beta blockers, calcium channel antagonists, and nitrates, especially in patients with chronic stable angina pectoris. Similar results have been noted in patients with CHF. In one double-blind study, only one month of treatment (500 mg three times daily) was necessary to cause significant improvement in heart function.[9] The longer carnitine was used, the more dramatic the improvement. After six months of use, the carnitine group demonstrated a 25.9% increase in the maximum exercise time and a 13.6% increase in ventricular ejection fraction. In another double-blind study in similar patients, at the end of six months of treatment, maximum exercise time on the treadmill increased 16.4% and the ejection fraction increased 12.1%.[10] Even more obvious benefits were seen in a three-year study of 80 patients with moderate to severe heart failure caused by a condition known as dilated cardiomyopathy.[11]

COENZYME Q_{10}

CoQ_{10} is another essential component of the mitochondria, where it plays a major role in energy production. Like carnitine, CoQ_{10} can be made within the body. Nonetheless, deficiencies have been reported. Deficiency can be a result of impaired CoQ_{10} production due to nutritional deficiencies, a genetic or acquired defect in CoQ_{10} synthesis (e.g., statin drugs block CoQ_{10} formation), or increased tissue needs.

Cardiovascular diseases, including angina, hypertension, mitral valve prolapse, and CHF, are examples of diseases that require increased tissue levels of CoQ_{10}. In addition, many elderly people may have increased CoQ_{10} requirements: The decline of CoQ_{10} levels that occurs with age may be partly responsible for the age-related deterioration of the immune system.

CoQ_{10} deficiency is common in individuals with heart disease. Heart tissue biopsies in patients with various heart diseases show a CoQ_{10} deficiency in 50–75% of cases. One of the most metabolically active tissues in the body, the heart may be unusually susceptible to the effects of CoQ_{10} deficiency. Accordingly, CoQ_{10} has shown great promise in the treatment of heart conditions. In one study, 12 patients with stable angina pectoris were treated with CoQ_{10} (150 mg/day for four weeks) in a double-blind, cross-over trial.[12] Compared with placebo, CoQ_{10} reduced the frequency of angina attacks by 53%. In addition, there was a significant increase in treadmill exercise tolerance (time to onset of chest pain and time to development of electrocardiogram abnormalities) during CoQ_{10} treatment. The results of this study and others suggest that CoQ_{10} is a safe and effective treatment for angina pectoris.

In the treatment of CHF, studies most often have used CoQ_{10} as a support aid (adjunct) to conventional drug therapy. The improvements noted with CoQ_{10} were actually found to be more positive than those obtained from conventional drug therapy alone in these studies.

In the largest study to date, 2,664 patients with mild to moderate CHF were enrolled in an open study in Italy.[13] The daily dosage of CoQ_{10} was 50–150 mg orally for 90 days, with the majority of patients (78%) receiving 100 mg/day. Table 7.1 shows the proportions of patients with improvement in clinical signs and symptoms after three months of CoQ_{10} treatment.

Table 7.1 Improvement in Congestive Heart Failure Symptoms with CoQ_{10}

Signs and Symptoms	Percent of Patients Showing Improvement
Sweating	79.8
Edema (fluid retention)	78.6
Cyanosis	78.1
Pulmonary edema	77.8
Heart palpitations	75.4
Vertigo	73.1
Venous congestion	71.8
Insomnia	66.2
Subjective arrhythmia	63.4
Nocturnal urination	53.6
Shortness of breath	52.7
Enlargement of liver area	49.3

Improvement of at least three symptoms occurred in 54% of patients, indicating a significantly improved quality of life with CoQ_{10} supplementation.

The results also showed a low incidence of side effects – only 36 patients (1.5%) reported mild side effects attributed to CoQ_{10}.

An important consideration in patients with CHF, especially more serious forms, is that they often fail to achieve adequate plasma CoQ_{10} levels (i.e., more than 2.5 mcg/ml) on supplemental ubiquinone (the common form of CoQ_{10}), even at dosages of up to 900 mg/day. These patients may respond better with highly absorbed forms of CoQ_{10}, such as ubiquinol or emulsified ubiquinone.

In one study, seven patients with advanced CHF with an average plasma CoQ_{10} level of 1.6 mcg/ml, taking an average dose of 450 mg of ubiquinone daily (150–600 mg/day), were changed to an average of 580 mg/day of ubiquinol (450–900 mg/day). Follow-up plasma CoQ_{10} levels, clinical status, and ejection fraction measurements done with echocardiography were studied.[14] Average plasma CoQ_{10} levels increased from 1.6 mcg/ml to 6.5 mcg/ml. The average ejection improved from 22% (range, 10–35%) to 39% (range, 10–60%). In this study, ubiquinol dramatically improved absorption in patients with severe heart failure and the improvement in plasma CoQ_{10} levels correlates with both clinical improvement and improvement in measurement of left ventricular function.

HAWTHORN *(CRATAEGUS OXYACANTHA)*

Hawthorn berry and flowering top extracts are widely used in Europe for their cardiovascular activity. They exhibit a combination of effects that are of great value to patients with angina and other heart problems. Studies have demonstrated that hawthorn extracts are effective in reducing angina attacks, lowering blood pressure and serum cholesterol levels, and improving heart function.[15-17]

The beneficial effects are due to improvement in the blood and oxygen supply of the heart resulting from dilation of the coronary vessels, as well as improvement of the metabolic processes in the heart.

Hawthorn's ability to dilate coronary blood vessels has been repeatedly demonstrated in experimental studies. In addition, hawthorn extracts have been shown to improve cardiac energy metabolism in human and experimental studies. This combined effect is extremely important in the treatment of angina because it results in improved myocardial function with more efficient use of oxygen. The improvement results not only from increased blood and oxygen supply to the heart muscle but also from hawthorn flavonoids interacting with key enzymes to enhance the heart's ability to contract properly.

CORONARY ANGIOGRAM, ANGIOPLASTY, AND ARTERY BYPASS SURGERY

An angiogram (cardiac catheterization) is an X-ray procedure in which dye is injected into the coronary arteries to locate blockages. These blockages are then most often opened with balloon angioplasty (a surgical procedure in which the diameter of the blocked artery is increased with the aid of a very small balloon attached to a flexible tube); the placement of a stent (a tiny wire mesh tube that acts as scaffolding to maintain and support the opening of an artery); and/or coronary artery bypass surgery (a procedure in which the coronary artery is bypassed by constructing an alternate route using a portion of a vein from the patient's leg). Patients often agree to these procedures without careful consideration of the risks and benefits.

These procedures – angiograms, bypass surgery, and angioplasty – are big business. Over one million heart angiograms are performed each year, for a total annual cost of over $10 billion. But based on extensive analysis, it appears that most of this money is wasted.

Several studies have challenged the widespread recommendation of angiograms made by most cardiologists.[18] One study evaluated 168 patients who were told they needed an angiogram to determine the degree of blockage, followed by bypass surgery or angioplasty. Using noninvasive tests, such as the exercise stress test, echocardiography (an ultrasound exam that measures the size and functional status of the heart), and the Holter monitor (a portable heart monitor worn for 24 hours to measure the pulse and characterize beats as normal or abnormal), the researchers determined that 134 of the patients, or 80%, did not need the catheterization.

Over a five-year period, this group of 168 patients had only a 1.1% rate of fatal heart attacks annually. This rate is much lower than the mortality rates associated with either coronary artery bypass surgery (5–10%) and no worse than that of angioplasty (1–2%). The researchers concluded that "in a large fraction of medically stable patients with coronary disease who are urged to undergo coronary angiography (heart catheterization), the procedure can be safely deferred." Noninvasive testing to determine the functional state of the heart is far more important in determining the type of therapy needed than the dangerous search for blocked arteries. If the heart is not functioning well, *then* the angiogram may be needed to see if surgery should be done.

Furthermore, the blockages found by the angiogram are usually not relevant to the patient's risk of heart attack. For instance, in the most sophisticated study of bypass surgery, the Coronary Artery Surgery Study (CASS), it was demonstrated that patients with healthy hearts but with one, two, or all three of the major heart vessels blocked did surprisingly well without surgery.[19–21] Regardless of the number or severity of the blockages, each group had the same low death rate of 1% per year.

That same year, the average death rate from bypass surgery was 10.1%, or about one death per 10 operations. In other words, the operation being recommended supposedly to save lives was 5–10 times more deadly than the disease. The best that can be said about bypass surgery and balloon angioplasty is that they are irrelevant to the course of the disease in all but the most serious cases. Patients who elect not to have the surgery live just as long as, or longer than, those who have the surgery.[22]

The severity of blockage does not necessarily correlate with reduction in blood flow in the artery. In one study, Iowa researchers measured blood flow in over 44 blockages demonstrated by angiogram.[23] Much to their surprise, they found no correlation between blood flow and the severity of the heart artery blockage. In other words, the angiogram did not provide clinically relevant information. The researchers found that "the coronary artery with a ninety-six-percent blockage had one of the most brisk blood flows, while a similar artery, with only forty-percent blockage, had severe blood-flow restriction." The authors concluded that the blockages found by heart catheterization simply do not correlate with blood-flow restriction. The researchers also commented that "the results of these studies should be profoundly disturbing.... . Information cannot be determined accurately by conventional angiographic approaches."

The bottom line is this: When patients are advised to have a coronary angiogram, chances are eight out of 10 that they do not need it. The critical factor in whether a patient needs coronary artery bypass surgery or angioplasty is how well the left ventricular pump is working, not the degree of blockage or the number of arteries affected. The left ventricle (chamber) of the heart is responsible for pumping oxygenated blood through the aorta (the large artery coming from the heart) and to the rest of the body. Bypass surgery is helpful only when the ejection fraction (the amount of blood pumped by the left ventricle) is less than 40% of capacity.[23] Up to 90% of all bypass procedures are done when the ejection fraction is greater than 50%, which is adequate for circulatory needs. In other words, as many as 90% of all bypass procedures may be unnecessary.

Angioplasty – or as it is known in research circles, percutaneous coronary intervention (PCI) – has largely replaced coronary artery bypass surgery. The results from large studies of angioplasty procedures, including the use of stents that release drugs to prevent blockage (drug-eluting stents), show the same lack of benefit as bypass operations. For example, the main results of the Clinical Outcomes Utilizing Revascularization and Aggressive DruG Evaluation (COURAGE) trial revealed no significant differences between PCI and medical therapy alone in the primary end point of all-cause mortality or non-fatal heart attacks, or in major secondary end points (composites of death/heart attack/stroke; hospitalization for angina or heart attacks) over a 4.6 year follow-up in 2,287 patients with stable coronary artery disease.[24]

When coronary artery bypass surgery or angioplasty is necessary, based on these accepted criteria, they definitely increase long-term survival and give relief of symptoms for 85% of patients. However, the surgery is not without risk. Complications arising from coronary bypass operations are common – this surgery is one of the most technically difficult procedures in modern medicine. Considering the cost of the procedure, the lack of long-term survival benefit, and the high level of complications, it appears that electing to have this surgery is unwise for the majority of patients.

This is particularly true in light of the availability of effective natural alternatives to coronary bypass surgery. Numerous studies have shown that dietary and lifestyle changes can significantly reduce the risk of heart attack and other causes of death due to atherosclerosis (hardening of the arteries). Simple dietary changes – decreasing the amount of saturated fat and cholesterol in the diet; increasing the consumption of dietary fiber, complex carbohydrates, fish oils, and magnesium; eliminating alcohol consumption and cigarette smoking; and reducing high blood pressure – would greatly reduce the number of coronary bypass operations performed in Westernized countries. In addition, clinical studies have shown that several nutritional supplements and botanical medicines improve heart function in even the most severe angina cases.

Another important alternative is intravenous EDTA chelation therapy (discussed below). Although this therapy is controversial, considerable clinical research has proven its efficacy.

WHEN AN ANGIOGRAM IS UNAVOIDABLE

When an angiogram or angioplasty is deemed necessary, the goal is then to prevent the damaging effects these procedures produce. This can be accomplished with a high-potency multivitamin and mineral formula, along with additional vitamin C (minimum 500 mg three times daily) and CoQ10 (300 mg daily two weeks prior to surgery and for three months afterward). It is generally recommended that garlic supplementation and high dosages of vitamin E (greater than 200 IU) be avoided prior to any surgery, owing to their ability to possibly promote excessive bleeding by inhibiting platelet aggregation – a key aspect of blood clot formation.

Vitamin C supplementation is rarely employed in hospitals, despite the fact that it may provide significant benefits; low vitamin C status is quite common in hospitalized patients. In a study analyzing the vitamin C status of patients undergoing coronary artery bypass, the plasma concentration of vitamin C was shown to plummet by 70% 24 hours after coronary artery bypass surgery; this level persisted in most patients for up to two weeks after surgery.[25] In contrast, vitamin E and carotene levels did not change to any significant degree, presumably because they are fat-soluble and are therefore retained in the body longer. Given the importance of vitamin C, the serious depletion of vitamin C may deteriorate defense mechanisms against free radicals and infection, and hinder wound repair, in these patients. Supplementation appears to be essential in patients recovering from heart surgery, or any surgery for that matter.

Return of blood flow (reperfusion) after coronary artery bypass surgery results in oxidative damage to the vascular endothelium and myocardium and thus greatly increases the risk of subsequent coronary artery disease. CoQ_{10} is recommended in an attempt to prevent such oxidative damage after bypass surgery or angioplasty. In one study, 40 patients undergoing elective surgery either served in the control group or received 150 mg of CoQ_{10} each day for seven days before the surgery.[26] The concentrations of lipid peroxides and the enzyme creatine kinase, which indicate myocardial damage, were significantly lower in patients who received CoQ_{10} than in the control group. The treatment group also showed a statistically significant lower incidence of ventricular arrhythmias during recovery. These results clearly demonstrate that pretreatment with CoQ_{10} can play a protective role during routine bypass surgery by reducing oxidative damage.

INTRAVENOUS ETHYLENEDIAMINETETRAACETIC ACID CHELATION THERAPY

Intravenous ethylenediaminetetraacetic acid (EDTA) chelation therapy is promoted as an alternative to coronary artery bypass surgery and angioplasty. EDTA is an amino-acid-like molecule that when slowly infused into the bloodstream binds with minerals such as calcium, iron, copper, and lead and carries them to the kidneys, where they are excreted. EDTA chelation has been commonly used to treat lead poisoning, but in the late 1950s and early 1960s it was found to help patients with atherosclerosis.

The discovery of EDTA chelation therapy as a treatment for angina and other conditions associated with atherosclerosis happened accidentally. In 1956 a battery worker whom Dr. Norman Clarke was treating with EDTA for lead poisoning noticed that his symptoms of angina disappeared. Clarke and others began using EDTA chelation therapy in patients with angina, cerebral vascular insufficiency, and occlusive peripheral vascular disease.

In a series of 283 patients treated by Clarke and his colleagues from 1956 to 1960, 87% showed improvements in their symptoms. Heart patients improved, and patients with blocked arteries in the legs, particularly those with diabetes, avoided amputation.[27,28]

It was originally thought that EDTA opened blocked arteries by chelating out the calcium deposits in the cholesterol plaque. However, its effectiveness now seems more related to chelating out excess iron and copper, minerals that, in the presence of oxygen, stimulate free radicals. Free radicals damage the cells in the artery and are a primary reason for atherosclerosis.

In a review of the progression and regression of atherosclerosis, the authors write that the process of atherosclerosis is "dependent on the presence of some metals (copper and iron) and can be completely inhibited by chelating agents such as EDTA."[29]

Despite obvious benefits to heart patients, EDTA fell out of favor in the mid-1960s. Advocates believe this occurred for two reasons: (1) the lucrative surgical approach to heart and vessel disease was on the rise and (2) the patent on EDTA held by Abbott Laboratories expired, so there was no financial interest for drug companies to fund any research.

Fortunately, in 1972 a small group of practicing physicians using EDTA chelation therapy founded an organization now called the American College for the Advancement of Medicine to continue education and research in this important area.

In the early days of EDTA chelation therapy, several serious problems were discovered. Giving too much EDTA or giving it too fast was soon noted to be dangerous. In fact, several deaths attributed to kidney failure were caused by EDTA toxicity. Fortunately, additional research resulted in more appropriate protocols, and EDTA chelation therapy as used now is safe. No deaths or significant adverse reactions have occurred in more than 500,000 patients who have undergone EDTA chelation therapy. Because EDTA chelation improves blood flow throughout the body, the side effects are usually beneficial and only a few adverse effects are noticed.

A substantial body of scientific evidence exists on the use of EDTA chelation therapy in the treatment of angina, peripheral vascular disease, and cerebral vascular disease.[30-34]

To clarify the benefits of EDTA chelation, the National Institutes of Health, including the National Heart, Lung, and Blood Institute and the National Center for Complementary and Alternative Medicine, sponsored the Trial to Assess Chelation Therapy, the first large-scale, multicenter study designed to determine the safety and efficacy of EDTA chelation therapy for individuals with coronary heart disease.[35] In the study, 839 subjects were randomized to receive EDTA infusions; 869 were randomized to receive placebo infusions. The results showed a slight advantage for chelation over placebo in the "primary composite endpoint," a combination of five separate outcomes: death, heart attack, stroke, coronary revascularization, and hospitalization for angina. These results are very encouraging and indicate that some patients experience the desired outcomes with EDTA chelation.

For more information, go to acam.org.

STROKE RECOVERY

A stroke is a vascular event that leads to brain damage. Strokes are the leading cause of adult disability in the United States and the third leading cause of death. A stroke can be the result of a lack of blood flow caused by blockage from a blood clot, or the result of a hemorrhage. Without oxygen, the brain cells become damaged or die, leaving the affected area of the brain unable to function. A stroke may result in an inability to move one or both limbs on one side of the body, inability to understand or formulate speech, or inability to see one side of the visual field. If the stroke is severe enough or occurs in a certain location, such as parts of the brainstem, it can result in coma or death.

In most cases, a stroke is a consequence of atherosclerosis. Risk factors for stroke include high blood pressure, previous stroke or transient ischemic attack (TIA, or "mini-stroke"), diabetes, high cholesterol, cigarette smoking, and atrial fibrillation (a heart abnormality). High blood pressure is by far the most important risk factor for a stroke.

MEDICAL CARE OF THE STROKE PATIENT

One of the key factors in limiting the damage to the brain caused by a stroke is how quickly a person receives medical treatment. The most effective conventional medical treatment uses the drug form of the naturally occurring compound tissue plasminogen activator (rTPA). It must be administered within a few hours of a stroke to produce significant benefit. Unfortunately, only 1–3% of stroke patients receive rTPA treatment.

The results of a stroke can affect patients physically, mentally, and emotionally – or in a combination of ways – and can vary widely depending on the size and location of the injury. Disability corresponds to the areas in the brain that have been damaged.

For most stroke patients who have post-stroke disability, recovery is a concerted effort that involves physical therapy, occupational therapy, and speech-language pathology. It is important to take advantage of all of these services because they can greatly aid the rehabilitation process.

Medical care often focuses on preventing another stroke and most often uses anti-coagulant therapy with warfarin (Coumadin) or anti-platelet therapy with aspirin or clopidogrel (Plavix), ticlopidine (Ticlid), or other drugs.

PRECAUTIONS WITH WARFARIN

The drug warfarin (Coumadin) works by blocking the action of vitamin K. Since green leafy vegetables and green tea contain high levels of vitamin K, these foods should be avoided while taking warfarin. However, most people can usually eat the same amounts they are accustomed to as long as they don't increase their consumption.

Physicians monitor the effects of warfarin using a test known as the international normalized ratio (INR) and will adjust the dosage up or down as needed. In addition to food high in vitamin K, other natural remedies may interact with warfarin, including the following:

- Coenzyme Q10 and St. John's wort (Hypericum perforatum) may reduce warfarin's efficacy.

- Several herbs, including Panax ginseng, devil's claw (Harpagophytum procumbens), and dong quai (Angelica sinensis), can increase warfarin's effects. It's likely that you can continue using these products, but don't change the dosage your body is accustomed to. INR values must be monitored appropriately.

- Garlic (Allium sativum) and ginkgo (Ginkgo biloba) extracts may reduce the ability of platelets to stick together, increasing the likelihood of bleeding. However, neither appears to interact directly with warfarin. Generally, people taking warfarin should avoid taking these products at higher dosages (more than the equivalent of one clove of garlic per day for garlic or more than 240 mg per day of ginkgo extract) but need not worry if they are taking just the typical support dose.

- Iron, magnesium, and zinc may bind with warfarin, potentially decreasing its absorption and activity. Take warfarin and products containing iron, magnesium, or zinc at least two hours apart.

- Nattokinase should not be used with warfarin unless INR levels are closely monitored.

To reduce the likelihood of bleeding and easy bruising with warfarin, consider taking 150–300 mg of either grape seed or pine bark extract daily.

These drugs are designed to prevent blood clots from forming and lodging in the brain, producing another stroke. These drugs are not, of course, used if the stroke was caused by a hemorrhage.

NATURAL PRODUCTS IN STROKE RECOVERY

From a natural perspective the goals are similar, but more focused on maximizing blood flow and nutrition to the damaged areas. In particular, nattokinase (see Chapter 1) and *Ginkgo biloba* extract are very important in stroke recovery. *Ginkgo biloba* extract increases blood flow to the brain, improves the production of energy within nerve cells, and favorably affects blood viscosity (thickness), resulting in improved blood flow characteristics within the brain. The recommended dosage is 240–320 mg daily.

In addition to nattokinase, a number of other dietary supplements can prevent blood clots from forming. These include omega-3 fatty acids, antioxidant nutrients, flavonoids, flavonoid-rich extracts (e.g., grape seed and pine bark extract), and garlic preparations standardized for alliin content. Fish oil supplementation (up to 3000 mg per day EPA+DHA) and flavonoid-rich extracts appear to be safe in combination with aspirin and other platelet inhibitors, but there may be issues if you are using several natural anti-platelet agents at the same time – doing so may increase bleeding tendencies when combined with anti-platelet drugs (including aspirin, but especially drugs like clopidogrel or ticlopidine).

Two highly bioavailable forms of the nutrient choline have shown effects in aiding stroke recovery: citicoline (also called CDP-choline) and glycerophosphocholine (GPC).[36] Of these, the research on GPC is a bit stronger. In six published clinical trials GPC has been given to almost 3,000 stroke patients.[36-41] The single largest trial included 2,044 patients.[38] At the end of the six-month trial, the investigators found that GPC significantly helped more than 95% of patients and was without side effects. Overall, GPC was judged by 78% of investigators as "very good" or "good," by 17% as "moderate," and by just 5% as having "poor" or "no" efficacy. Choose either citocoline

1000–2000 mg daily or GPC 600–1200 mg daily. There are no known interactions between citocoline or GPC and warfarin or anti-platelet drugs.

FINAL COMMENTS

Let me put things in focus by consolidating the supplement recommendations for angina, CHF, arrhythmias, and other heart ailments.

NUTRITIONAL SUPPLEMENTS

- High-potency multivitamin and mineral supplement according to guidelines given in Chapter 2
- Key individual nutrients:
  - Vitamin C: 500–1000 mg daily
  - Magnesium, preferably bound to aspartate, citrate, or other Krebs cycle intermediate: 150–250 mg 2–3 times daily
- Fish oils: 3000 mg EPA+DHA daily
- Choose one of the following:
  - Grape seed extract (more than 95% procyanidolic oligomers): 150–300 mg daily
  - Pine bark extract (more than 90% procyanidolic oligomers): 150–300 mg daily
- Carnitine: 500 mg three times daily
- Pantethine: 300 mg three times daily
- Coenzyme Q_{10}: 100 mg 2–3 times daily (in more severe cases, consider ubiquinol or $BioQ_{10}$ SA – a highly bioavailable form of CoQ_{10} – for enhanced absorption)

BOTANICAL MEDICINES

- Hawthorn *(Crataegus oxyacantha)* extract standardized to contain 10% procyanidins or 1.8% vitexin-4'-rhamnoside: 100–250 mg three times daily

RESOURCES

APPENDIX A – **DIETARY FIBER CONTENT OF SELECTED FOODS**

Food	Serving	Calories	Grams of Fiber
FRUIT			
Apple (with skin)	1 medium	81	3.5
Banana	1 medium	105	2.4
Cantaloupe	¼ melon	30	1.0
Cherries, sweet	10	49	1.2
Grapefruit	½ medium	38	1.6
Orange	1 medium	62	2.6
Peach (with skin)	1 medium	37	1.9
Pear (with skin)	½ large	61	3.1
Prunes	3	60	3.0
Raisins	¼ cup	106	3.1
Raspberries	½ cup	35	3.1
Strawberries	1 cup	45	3.0
VEGETABLES, RAW			
Bean sprouts	½ cup	13	1.5
Celery, diced	½ cup	10	1.1
Cucumber	½ cup	8	0.4
Lettuce	1 cup	10	0.9

Food	Serving	Calories	Grams of Fiber
Mushrooms	½ cup	10	1.5
Pepper, green	½ cup	9	0.5
Spinach	1 cup	8	1.2
Tomato	1 medium	20	1.5
VEGETABLES, COOKED			
Asparagus, cut	1 cup	30	2.0
Beans, green	1 cup	32	3.2
Broccoli	1 cup	40	4.4
Brussels sprouts	1 cup	56	4.6
Cabbage, red	1 cup	30	2.8
Carrots	1 cup	48	4.6
Cauliflower	1 cup	28	2.2
Corn	½ cup	87	2.9
Kale	1 cup	44	2.8
Parsnip	1 cup	102	5.4
Potato (with skin)	1 medium	106	2.5
Potato (without skin)	1 medium	97	1.4
Spinach	1 cup	42	4.2
Sweet potatoes	1 medium	160	3.4
Zucchini	1 cup	22	3.6
LEGUMES			
Baked beans	½ cup	155	8.8
Dried peas, cooked	½ cup	115	4.7
Kidney beans, cooked	½ cup	110	7.3
Lentils, cooked	½ cup	97	3.7
Lima beans, cooked	½ cup	64	4.5
Navy beans, cooked	½ cup	112	6.0
RICE, BREADS, PASTAS			
Bran muffin	1 muffin	104	2.5

Food	Serving	Calories	Grams of Fiber
Bread, white	1 slice	78	0.4
Bread, whole wheat	1 slice	61	1.4
Crisp bread, rye	2 crackers	50	2.0
Rice, brown, cooked	½ cup	97	1.0
Rice, white, cooked	½ cup	82	0.2
Spaghetti, reg., cooked	½ cup	155	1.1
Spaghetti, whole wheat, cooked	½ cup	155	3.9
BREAKFAST CEREALS			
All Bran	⅓ cup	71	8.5
Bran Chex	⅔ cup	91	4.6
Corn Bran	⅔ cup	98	5.4
Corn flakes	1¼ cup	110	0.3
Grape-Nuts	¼ cup	101	1.4
Oatmeal	¾ cup	108	1.6
Raisin Bran-type	⅔ cup	115	4.0
Shredded Wheat	⅔ cup	102	2.6
NUTS			
Almonds	10 nuts	79	1.1
Filberts	10 nuts	54	0.8
Peanuts	10 nuts	105	1.4

APPENDIX B – GLYCEMIC INDEX, CARBOHYDRATE CONTENT, AND GLYCEMIC LOAD OF SELECTED FOODS

A complete list of the glycemic index and glycemic load of all tested foods is beyond the scope of this book – it would be a book in itself. So I have selected the most common foods. This listing will give you a general sense of high GL and low GL foods. We have listed the items by food groups, from low to high glycemic loads. You may notice that certain food groups are not listed. For example, you won't see nuts, seeds, fish, poultry, and meats listed because these foods have little impact on blood sugar levels because they are low in carbohydrates.

If you would like to see an even more complete listing, visit mendosa.com – it's a free website operated by medical writer Rick Mendosa and an excellent resource.

FOOD	GI	Carbs g	Fiber g	GL
BEANS (LEGUMES)				
Soybeans, cooked, ½ cup, 100 g	14	12	7	1.6
Peas, green, fresh, frozen, boiled, ½ cup, 80 g	48	5	2	2
White navy beans, boiled, ½ cup, 90 g	38	11	6	4.2
Kidney beans, boiled, ½ cup, 90 g	27	18	7.3	4.8
Peas, split, yellow, boiled, ½ cup, 90 g	32	16	4.7	5.1
Lentils, ½ cup, 100 g	28	19	3.7	5.3
Lima beans, baby, ½ cup cooked, 85 g	32	17	4.5	5.4
Black beans, canned, ½ cup, 95 g	45	15	7	5.7
Pinto beans, canned, ½ cup, 95 g	45	13	6.7	5.8

FOOD	GI	Carbs g	Fiber g	GL
Chickpeas, canned, drained, ½ cup, 95 g	42	15	5	6.3
Kidney beans, canned and drained, ½ cup, 95 g	52	13	7.3	6.7
Broad, frozen, boiled, ½ cup, 80 g	79	9	6	7.1
Peas, dried, boiled, ½ cup, 70 g	22	4	4.7	8
Baked beans, canned in tomato sauce, ½ cup, 120 g	48	21	8.8	10
Blackeyed beans, soaked, boiled, ½ cup, 120 g	42	24	5	10
BREAD				
Multigrain, unsweetened, 1 slice, 30 g	43	9	1.4	4
Oat bran & honey, 1 slice, 40 g	31	14	1.5	4.5
Sourdough, rye, 1 slice, 30 g	48	12	0.4	6
Stoneground whole wheat, 1 slice, 30 g	53	11	1.4	6
Wonder, enriched white bread, 1 slice, 20 g	73	10	0.4	7
Sourdough, wheat, 1 slice, 30 g	54	14	0.4	7.5
Pumpernickel, 1 slice, 60 g	41	21	0.5	8.6
Whole wheat, 1 slice, 35 g	69	14	1.4	9.6
Healthy Choice, hearty 7-grain, 1 slice, 38 g	56	18	1.4	10
White (wheat flour), 1 slice, 30 g	70	15	0.4	10.5
Healthy Choice, 100% whole grain, 1 slice, 38 g	62	18	1.4	11
Gluten-free multigrain, 1 slice, 35 g	79	15	1.8	12
French baguette, 30 g	95	15	0.4	14
Hamburger bun, 1 prepacked bun, 50 g	61	24	0.5	15
Rye, 1 slice, 50 g	65	23	0.4	15
Light rye, 1 slice, 50 g	68	23	0.4	16
Dark rye, Black, 1 slice, 50 g	76	21	0.4	16
Croissant, 1, 50 g	67	27	0.2	18
Kaiser roll, 1 roll, 50 g	73	25	0.4	18
Pita, 1 piece, 65 g	57	38	0.4	22
Bagel, 1, 70 g	72	35	0.4	25
BREAKFAST CEREALS				
Oat bran, raw, 1 tablespoon, 10 g	55	7	1	4
Bran with psyllium, ⅓ cup, 30 g	47	12	12.5	5.6
Bran, ⅓ cup, 30 g	58	14	14	8
All-Bran Soy n Fiber, ½ cup, 45 g	33	26	7	8.5
All-Bran, ½ cup, 40 g	42	22	6.5.	9.2
Oatmeal (cooked with water), 1 cup, 245 g	42	24	1.6	10

FOOD	GI	Carbs g	Fiber g	GL
Shredded wheat, ⅓ cup, 25 g	67	18	1.2	12
Mini Wheats (whole wheat), 1 cup, 30 g	58	21	4.4	12
All-Bran Fruit n Oats, ½ cup, 45 g	39	33	6	13
Weet-Bix, 2 biscuits, 30 g	69	19	2	13
Cheerios, ½ cup, 30 g	74	20	2	15
Frosties, ¾ cup, 30 g	55	27	1	15
Corn Bran, ½ cup, 30 g	75	20	1	15
Honey Smacks, ¾ cup, 30 g	56	27	1	15
Wheatbites, 30 g	72	22	2	16
Total, 30 g	76	22	2	16.7
Healthwise for heart health, 45 g	48	35	2	16.8
Mini Wheats (blackcurrant), 1 cup, 30 g	71	24	2	17
Puffed wheat, 1 cup, 30 g	80	22	2	17.6
Bran Flakes, ¾ cup, 30 g	74	24	2	18
Crunchy Nut Cornflakes (Kellogg's), 30 g	72	25	2	18
Froot Loops, 1 cup, 30 g	69	27	1	18
Cocoa Pops, ¾ cup, 30 g	77	26	1	20
Team, 30 g	82	25	1	20.5
Corn Chex, 30 g	83	25	1	20.75
Just Right, ¾ cup, 30 g	60	36	2	21.6
Corn Flakes, 1 cup, 30 g	84	26	0.3	21.8
Rice Krispies, 1 cup, 30 g	82	27	0.3	22
Rice Chex, 1 cup, 30 g	89	25	1	22
Crispix, 30 g	87	26	1	22.6
Just Right Just Grains, 1 cup, 45 g	62	38	2	23.5
Oat n Honey Bake, 45 g	77	31	2	24
Raisin Bran, 1 cup, 45 g	73	35	4	25.5
Grape-Nuts, ½ cup, 58 g	71	47	2	33.3
CAKE				
Cake, angel food, 1 slice, 30 g	67	17	<1	11.5
Cake, sponge cake, 1 slice, 60 g	46	32	<1	14.7
Cake, cupcake, with icing and cream filling, 1 cake, 38 g	73	26	<1	19
Cake, chocolate fudge, mix, (Betty Crocker), 73 g cake + 33 g frosting	38	54	<1	20.5
Cake, banana cake, 1 slice, 80 g	47	46	<1	21.6
Cake, pound cake, 1 slice, 80 g	54	42	<1	22.6

FOOD	GI	Carbs g	Fiber g	GL
Cake, French vanilla, (Betty Crocker), 73 g cake + 33 g frosting	42	58	<1	24.4
Cake, Lamingtons, 1, 50 g	87	29	<1	25
Cake, flan, 1 slice, 80 g	65	55	<1	35.75
Cake, scones, made from packet mix, 1 scone, 40 g	92	90	<1	83
CRACKERS				
Crackers, Corn Thins, puffed corn, 2, 12 g	87	9	<1	7.8
Crackers, Kavli, 4, 20 g	71	13	3	9.2
Crackers, Breton wheat crackers, 6, 25 g	67	14	2	9.4
Crackers, Ryvita or Wasa, 2, 20 g	69	16	3	11
Crackers, Stoned Wheat Thins, 5, 25 g	67	17	1	11.4
Crackers, Premium soda crackers, 3, 25 g	74	17	0	12.5
Crackers, water cracker, 5, 25 g	78	18	0	14
Crackers, graham 1, 30 g	74	22	1.4	16
Crackers, rice cake, 2, 25 g	82	21	0.4	17
MILK, SOY MILK, AND JUICES				
Milk, full fat, 1 cup, 250 ml	27	12	0	3
Soy, 1 cup, 250 ml	31	12	0	3.7
Milk, skim, 1 cup, 250 ml	32	13	0	4
Grapefruit juice, unsweetened, 1 cup, 250 ml	48	16	1	7.7
Nesquik chocolate powder, 3 tsp in 250 ml milk	55	14	0	7.7
Milk, chocolate flavored, low fat, 1 cup, 250 ml	34	23	0	7.8
Orange juice, 1 cup, 250 ml	46	21	1	9.7
Gatorade, 1 cup, 250 ml	78	15	0	11.7
Pineapple juice, unsweetened, canned, 250 ml	46	27	1	12.4
Apple juice, unsweetened, 1 cup, 250 ml	40	33	1	13.2
Cranberry juice cocktail (Ocean Spray USA), 240 ml	68	34	0	23
Coca Cola, 375 ml	63	40	0	25.2
Soft drinks, 375 ml	68	51	0	34.7
Milk, sweetened condensed, ½ cup, 160 g	61	90	0	55
FRUIT				
Cherries, 20 cherries, 80 g	22	10	2.4	2.2
Plums, 3–4 small, 100 g	39	7	2.2	2.7
Peach, fresh, 1 large, 110 g	42	7	1.9	3
Apricots, fresh, 3 medium, 100 g	57	7	1.9	4
Apricots, dried, 5–6 pieces, 30 g	31	13	2.2	4

FOOD	GI	Carbs g	Fiber g	GL
Kiwi, 1 raw, peeled, 80 g	52	8	2.4	4
Orange, 1 medium, 130 g	44	10	2.6	4.4
Peach, canned, in natural juice, ½ cup, 125 g	38	12	1.5	4.5
Pear, canned, in pear juice, ½ cup, 125 g	43	13	1.5	5.5
Watermelon, 1 cup, 150 g	72	8	1	5.7
Pineapple, fresh, 2 slices, 125 g	66	10	2.8	6.6
Apple, 1 medium, 150 g	38	18	3.5	6.8
Grapes, green, 1 cup, 100 g	46	15	2.4	6.9
Apple, dried, 30 g	29	24	3.0	6.9
Prunes, pitted (Sunsweet), 6 prunes, 40 g	29	25	3.0	7.25
Pear, fresh, 1 medium, 150 g	38	21	3.1	8
Fruit cocktail, canned in natural juice, ½ cup, 125 g	55	15	1.5	8.25
Apricots, canned, light syrup, ½ cup, 125 g	64	13	1.5	8.3
Peach, canned, light syrup, ½ cup, 125 g	52	18	1.5	9.4
Mango, 1 small, 150 g	55	19	2.0	10.4
Figs, dried, tenderized (water added), 50 g	61	22	3.0	13.4
Sultanas, ¼ cup, 40 g	56	30	3.1	16.8
Banana, raw, 1 medium, 150 g	55	32	2.4	17.6
Raisins, ¼ cup, 40 g	64	28	3.1	18
Dates, dried, 5, 40 g	103	27	3.0	27.8
GRAINS				
Rice bran, extruded, 1 tbsp, 10 g	19	3	1	0.57
Barley, pearled, boiled, ½ cup, 80 g	25	17	6	4.25
Millet, cooked, ½ cup, 120 g	71	12	1	8.52
Bulgur, cooked, ⅔ cup, 120 g	48	22	3.5	10.6
Brown rice, steamed, 1 cup, 150 g	50	32	1	16
Couscous, cooked, ⅔ cup, 120 g	65	28	1	18
Rice, white, boiled, 1 cup, 150 g	72	36	0.2	26
Rice, Arborio risotto rice, white, boiled, 100 g	69	35	0.2	29
Rice, basmati, white, boiled, 1 cup, 180 g	58	50	0.2	29
Buckwheat, cooked, ½ cup, 80 g	54	57	3.5	30
Rice, instant, cooked, 1 cup, 180 g	87	38	0.2	33
Tapioca (steamed 1 hour), 100 g	70	54	<1	38
Tapioca (boiled with milk), 1 cup, 265 g	81	51	<1	41
Rice, jasmine, white, long grain, steamed, 1 cup, 180 g	109	39	0.2	42.5

FOOD	GI	Carbs g	Fiber g	GL
ICE CREAM				
Ice cream, low-fat French vanilla, 100 ml	38	15	0	5.7
Ice cream, full fat, 2 scoops, 50 g	61	10	0	6.1
JAM				
Jam, no sugar, 1 tbsp, 25 g	55	11	<1	6
Jam, sweetened 1 tbsp	48	17	<1	8
MUFFINS AND PANCAKES				
Muffins, chocolate butterscotch, from mix, 50 g	53	28	1	15
Muffins, apple, oat and sultana, from mix, 50 g	54	28	1	15
Muffins, apricot, coconut and honey, from mix, 50 g	60	27	1.5	16
Muffins, banana, oat and honey, from mix, 50 g	65	28	1.5	18
Muffins, apple, 1 muffin, 80 g	44	44	1,5	19
Muffins, bran, 1 muffin, 80 g	60	34	2.5	20
Muffins, blueberry, 1 muffin, 80 g	59	41	1,5	24
Pancake, buckwheat, from dry mix, 40 g	102	30	2	30
Pancake, from dry mix, 1 large, 80 g	67	58	1	39
PASTA				
Pasta, tortellini, cheese, cooked, 180 g	50	21	2	10.5
Pasta, ravioli, meat-filled, cooked, 1 cup, 220 g	39	30	2	11.7
Pasta, vermicelli, cooked, 1 cup, 180 g	35	45	2	15.7
Pasta, rice noodles, fresh, boiled, 1 cup, 176 g	40	44	0.4	17.6
Pasta, spaghetti, whole meal, cooked, 1 cup, 180 g	37	48	3.5	17.75
Pasta, fettuccine, cooked, 1 cup, 180 g	32	57	2	18.2
Pasta, spaghetti, gluten free, in tomato sauce, 1 small tin, 220 g	68	27	2	18.5
Pasta, macaroni and cheese, packaged, cooked, 220 g	64	30	2	19.2
Pasta, Star Pastina, cooked, 1 cup, 180 g	38	56	2	21
Pasta, spaghetti, white, cooked, 1 cup, 180 g	41	56	2	23
Pasta, rice pasta, brown, cooked, 1 cup, 180 g	92	57	2	52
SUGARS				
Fructose, 10 g	23	10	0	2.3
Honey, ½ tablespoon, 10 g	58	16	0	4.6
Lactose, 10 g	46	10	0	4.6
Sucrose, 10 g	65	10	0	6.5
Glucose, 10 g	102	10	0	10.2
Maltose, 10 g	105	10	0	10.5

FOOD	GI	Carbs g	Fiber g	GL
SNACKS				
Corn chips, Doritos original, 50 g	42	33	<1	13.9
Snickers, 59 g	41	35	0	14.3
Tofu frozen dessert (non-dairy), 100 g	115	13	<1	15
Real Fruit bars, strawberry, 20 g	90	17	<1	15.3
Twix cookie bar (caramel), 59 g	44	37	<1	16.2
Pretzels, 50 g	83	22	<1	18.3
Mars bar, 60 g	65	41	0	26.6
Skittles, 62 g	70	55	0	38.5
SOUPS				
Tomato, canned, 220 ml	38	15	1.5	6
Black bean, 220 ml	64	9	3.4	6
Lentil, canned, 220 ml	44	14	3	6
Split pea, canned, 220 ml	60	13	3	8
VEGETABLES				
Carrots, raw, ½ cup, 80 g	16	6	1.5	1
Carrots, peeled, boiled, ½ cup, 70 g	49	3	1.5	1.5
Beets, canned, drained, 2–3 slices, 60 g	64	5	1	3
Pumpkin, peeled, boiled, ½ cup, 85 g	75	6	3.4	4.5
Parsnips, boiled, ½ cup, 75 g	97	8	3	8
Sweet corn on the cob, boiled 20 min, 80 g	48	14	2.9	8
Corn, canned and drained, ½ cup, 80 g	55	15	3	8.5
Sweet potato, peeled, boiled, 80 g	54	16	3.4	8.6
Sweet corn, ½ cup boiled, 80 g	55	18	3	10
Potatoes, peeled, boiled, 1 medium, 120 g	87	13	1.4	10
Potatoes, with skin, boiled, 1 medium, 120 g	79	15	2.4	11
Yam, boiled, 80 g	51	26	3.4	13
Potatoes, baked in oven (no fat), 1 medium, 120 g	93	15	2.4	14
Potatoes, mashed, ½ cup, 120 g	91	16	1	14
Potatoes, Instant potato, prepared, ½ cup	83	18	1	15
Potatoes, new, unpeeled, boiled, 5 small (cocktail), 175 g	78	25	2	20
Cornmeal (polenta), ⅓ cup, 40 g	68	30	2	20
Potatoes, French fries, fine cut, small serving, 120 g	75	49	1	36
Gnocchi, cooked, 1 cup, 145 g	68	71	1	48

FOOD	GI	Carbs g	Fiber g	GL
LOW GLYCEMIC VEGETABLES				
Asparagus, 1 cup, cooked or raw Bell Peppers, 1 cup, cooked or raw Broccoli, 1 cup, cooked or raw Brussels sprouts, 1 cup, cooked or raw Cabbage, 1 cup, cooked or raw Cauliflower, 1 cup, cooked or raw Cucumber, 1 cup Celery, 1 cup, cooked or raw Eggplant, 1 cup Green beans, 1 cup, cooked or raw Kale, 1 cup cooked, 2 cups raw Lettuce, 2 cups raw Mushrooms, 1 cup Spinach, 1 cup cooked, 2 cups raw Tomatoes, 1 cup Zucchini, 1 cup, cooked or raw	≈20	≈7	≈1.5	≈1.4
YOGURT				
Yogurt, low fat, artificial sweetener, 200 g	14	12	0	2
Yogurt, with fruit, 200 g	26	30	0	8
Yogurt, low fat, 200 g	33	26	0	8.5

APPENDIX C – **FREQUENTLY ASKED QUESTIONS ON PGX®**

WHAT IS PGX®?

PGX® (PolyGlycopleX®) is a unique complex of highly purified, water-soluble dietary fiber developed using advanced EnviroSimplex® technology. This technology combines these natural compounds in a very specific ratio making PGX® an effective weight loss aid and dietary supplement. PGX® was invented by researchers at InovoBiologic Inc., Calgary after many years of extensive research. PGX® is available in a variety of forms including capsules, soft gelatin capsules, granules, meal replacement powders, and pre-meal drink mixes.

WHERE CAN I BUY PGX®?

PGX® products are available under a variety of brand names, in stores throughout North America that sell natural health products. Visit pgx.com and select "Where to Buy" under the "About PGX®" main menu, enter an address, and click the "Find Nearest" button to see the nearest locations.

WHAT IS THE PGX® DAILY ULTRA MATRIX TECHNOLOGY?

PGX® technology has produced PGX® Daily Ultra Matrix Softgels – an advanced delivery system for optimum results. "Ultra Matrix" refers to PGX® granules suspended in a matrix of medium chain triglycerides (MCTs) – healthy fats from purified coconut oil. PGX® Daily disperses and becomes viscous slowly in the stomach and digestive tract. Most other fibers do not become as viscous as PGX®, become viscous too quickly, or do not become viscous at all. PGX®

maintains its viscosity throughout the entire digestive tract (including the colon) which means that the glycemic index and subsequent blood sugar regulation is greater. Also, thanks to the thermogenic properties of the MCTs in the capsule, PGX® Daily can result in an extra 25–50 calories burned daily.

HOW DO I USE PGX®?

To enjoy the full benefits of PGX®, try to take some before each and every meal. Be sure to drink at least 250 ml (8 oz) of water per 2.5 gram serving of PGX®. Start with 1–2 softgels of PGX® Daily before each meal and increase by 1 softgel per meal every 2–3 days. If you are prone to digestive upset, increase the dose at a slower rate to give your body time to adjust. Some people find 2–3 softgels or 2.5 grams of PGX® granules to be effective. Others require the maximum dose of 6 softgels of PGX® Daily or 5 grams of PGX® granules in order to reduce portion size. Continue to increase the dosage until you experience a significant reduction in hunger and between-meal food cravings. Do not exceed 6 softgels or 5 grams up to three times per day.

DOES PGX® HAVE SIDE EFFECTS?

PGX® is a highly concentrated and highly effective form of fiber. It can take time for your body to adjust. To avoid minor side effects, such as increased gas, bloating, loose stools or constipation, it is best to start with small amounts of PGX® and then gradually increase your intake as your body adjusts. If you take PGX® consistently, and increase the dose gradually, it is likely that you will be able to consume a highly effective dose, without these effects, within a few days to a week. To decrease any possible side effects, it is important to drink a large glass of water with each dose of PGX®.

CAN PGX® BE TAKEN WITH MY MEDICATION?

PGX® can slow the rate of absorption of food and therefore it can theoretically do the same with medication. It is recommended that any oral medication be taken 1 hour before PGX® and/or 2–3 hours after consuming PGX® products. People with diabetes must monitor their blood glucose carefully as they may need to adjust medications accordingly. As PGX® helps control blood glucose, it may lessen the need for insulin or other medications over time. If you are on any medication consult a health care practitioner prior to using dietary supplements or changing your nutritional regimen.

CAN I TAKE PGX® WITH OTHER SUPPLEMENTS?

There is no problem taking PGX® along with supplements including essential fatty acids (EFAs) and multivitamins/multiminerals. A 21-day double-blind, placebo-controlled human tolerance study where 10 g of PGX® were given per day showed no statistical difference between levels of minerals and fat- and water-soluble vitamins in the test and control groups.

HOW FAST CAN I EXPECT TO LOSE WEIGHT?

Participants in a study who exercised and followed a 1,200 calorie/day diet lost on average 1–2 lbs per week. This is considered healthy weight loss. For some people weight loss is not immediate, while many people lose more weight depending upon their consistent use of PGX® and other lifestyle factors. PGX® makes following a calorie-restricted diet easy because it controls appetite due to its water solubility (absorbs many times its weight in water) and its ability to reduce and diminish cravings for starchy and sugary foods.

It is important to differentiate between weight loss and fat loss. As fat weighs less than muscle tissue, many people actually experience weight gain when they begin a reducing regime. Also, for some people, the additional water they drink with PGX® can temporarily add weight, since a liter of water weighs 1 kg or 2.2 lbs. While fast weight loss may seem ideal, it is important to remember that we gain weight gradually over a period of time. Losing weight the same way is "healthy weight loss" and will help reduce the risk of regaining the lost weight.

HOW DO I KNOW PGX® IS WORKING?
HOW MUCH DO I HAVE TO USE TO LOSE WEIGHT?

It is recommended that you start with a lower dose of PGX® for the first 3–7 days to see how your body adjusts to the increase in fiber intake. An increased amount of PGX®, to its active dosage (10–15 grams per day or 2.5–5 grams per meal) will produce noticeable reductions in appetite and cravings. Many people who have just started taking PGX® feel energized and notice their clothes fit better even though they have not changed anything else except taking PGX® everyday.

IF PGX® IS FIBER HOW CAN I GET CONSTIPATED?

PGX® can only cause constipation if your water intake is not adequate for the amount of PGX® you are consuming. PGX® expands to hold many times its weight in water. You need to drink at least 250 ml (8 oz) of water per 2.5 grams (2–3 softgels). It is also important to eat smaller amounts of food regularly and take PGX® according to label directions. Be sure to take in adequate fresh water – not drinks such as coffee or alcohol that can cause you to lose water. During the day you may want to drink non-caffeinated herbal teas, vegetable juice, or diluted fruit juice (watch the sugar content of juices). Also, be sure to take PGX® consistently. Do not skip days and, if you are prone to constipation, take PGX® at the same time every day.

WHAT CAN I DO ABOUT GAS AND BLOATING?

Reduce the amount of PGX® you are taking and once you feel comfortable (no gas or bloating) gradually increase the amount over a few days (3–7 days). These side effects are temporary with most people and completely subside after a week or more of use. You may also want to take probiotic supplements (friendly intestinal bacteria) to enhance the health of your gastrointestinal tract.

AFTER TAKING PGX® IS IT POSSIBLE TO STILL BE HUNGRY?

For some people, yes. One explanation is that when blood sugar has been out of control or imbalanced for a long time, and the body has not been using insulin properly, the brain can still send out powerful messages to eat. When you take PGX® every day these strong messages become weaker. The inappropriate messages to eat are no longer needed when blood sugar becomes balanced and the brain is satisfied it will get the glucose required to function.

I'VE TRIED OTHER DIETS. HOW IS PGX® DIFFERENT?

PGX® isn't a diet, but it can make any weight loss plan or diet work better. Research has shown that people who gain weight and have difficulty losing weight, often spend much of their day on a "blood sugar roller coaster" with blood sugar alternately surging and plummeting, leaving them tired or irritable and leading to frequent and unhealthy food cravings. PGX® helps re-train your body and eliminate the blood sugar roller coaster so you don't crave "bad foods" and so you can better control your appetite. With PGX® you can achieve lasting results.

HOW DOES PGX® CONTROL CRAVINGS?

Often blood sugar levels can make our bodies crave sugar and starchy foods. Blood sugar levels rise and fall naturally, but rapid changes are harmful and create many of the cravings we experience. When blood sugar levels drop, our brain tells us to eat and often we look for foods with lots of sugars, fats, and starches in order to raise sugar levels. By balancing blood sugar levels, the brain is no longer demanding fast energy and you will be less likely to crave food.

DOES PGX® CONTAIN GLUTEN?

PGX® softgels and PGX® granules are wheat and gluten free. PGX® meal replacement and pre-meal drink mix products cannot be considered gluten or wheat free.

DOES PGX® CONTAIN CAFFEINE OR OTHER STIMULANTS?

No. PGX® is a natural, non-addictive dietary supplement containing no caffeine or other stimulants.

HOW DO I KNOW IF MY BLOOD SUGAR IS "OUT OF BALANCE"?

Your doctor can do tests to determine whether or not your blood sugar levels are within normal range. The indicators you can see and feel yourself include:

- Cravings – especially sweets and carbohydrates.
- Feeling tired and irritable for no apparent reason.
- Gaining weight in spite of an unchanged diet or lifestyle.
- Feeling hungry again shortly after eating.

HOW DOES PGX® LOWER THE GLYCEMIC INDEX OF MEALS AND WHY IS THIS IMPORTANT?

Glycemic Index (GI) is a way of indicating how fast a particular food is turned into energy by the body. High GI foods are digested quickly and raise blood sugar fast. Low GI foods are converted to glucose more slowly. PGX® slows down the rate at which all food is digested, lowering after-meal blood sugar and virtually lowering the glycemic index of any food. Clinical studies show that high after-meal blood sugar levels are a major factor for heart disease risk.

HOW LONG DOES A PERSON HAVE TO TAKE PGX®?

After initial weight loss goals have been achieved, a lower "maintenance" dose of PGX® can effectively help control weight, appetite, blood sugar, and cholesterol for life. PGX® is non-habit forming but many people find that its effects – increased self esteem, a healthy weight, and more energy – are quite "addictive".

WHAT RESEARCH IS THERE TO SUPPORT THE BENEFITS AND EFFECTIVENESS OF PGX®?

PGX® is the result of many years of intensive clinical and laboratory research with universities from around the world and specialized research organizations in collaboration with the Canadian Centre for Functional Medicine. After years of research involving thousands of participants it is clear that adding PGX® to meals can: balance blood sugar, reduce the glycemic index of foods, restore insulin sensitivity (a key factor in weight control), curb food cravings, and lower cholesterol levels.

IS PGX® SUITABLE FOR CHILDREN?

Yes. Half the adult dose is recommended for children 9 years of age and older, or 1–3 softgels before each meal until the child notices a reduction in hunger and between-meal food cravings. However, children have unique developmental nutritional requirements. PGX® suppresses appetite and you should consult a qualified health care practitioner before giving PGX® to your child.

WHO SHOULD NOT USE PGX®?

Anyone who cannot compensate for a large water intake, such as someone with renal disease or congestive heart failure.

Anyone taking a large number of medications that must be taken with food and/or without food, unless advised by a health care practitioner.

Anyone who has difficulty swallowing, including people with gastrointestinal disorders and those with esophageal stenosis, or pre-existing bowel abnormalities, may be at risk for esophageal or intestinal blockages or obstruction and should consult a health care practitioner prior to use.

Pregnant or lactating women should discuss PGX® use with a health care practitioner prior to use.

Anyone under 18 years of age should discuss PGX® use with a health care practitioner prior to use.

If you have any concerns, consult a health care practitioner.

For more information on PGX® visit pgx.com

REFERENCES

The references provided are by no means designed to represent a complete reference list for all of the studies reviewed or mentioned in this book. In fact, I have chosen to focus on key studies and comprehensive review articles that readers, especially medical professionals, may find helpful.

CHAPTER 1 – THE HEART OF THE MATTER IS THE MATTER OF THE HEART

1 Khaw KT, Wareham N, Bingham S, et al. Combined impact of health behaviours and mortality in men and women: the EPIC-Norfolk prospective population study. *PLoS Med*. 2008 Jan 8;5(1):e12.

2 Elliot WJ. Ear lobe crease and coronary artery disease, 1,000 patients and a review of the literature. *Am J Med*. 1983;75(6):1024-32.

3 Elliott WJ, Powell LH. Diagonal earlobe creases and prognosis in patients with suspected coronary artery disease. *Am J Med*. 1996;100(2):205-11.

4 Qiao Q, Tervahauta M, Nissinen A, et al. Mortality from all causes and from coronary heart disease related to smoking and changes in smoking during a 35-year follow-up of middle-aged Finnish men. *Eur Heart J*. 2000;21(19):1621-6.

5 Levenson J, Simon AC, Cambien FA, et al. Cigarette smoking and hypertension. Factors independently associated with blood hyperviscosity and arterial rigidity. *Arteriosclerosis*. 1987;7(6):572-7.

6 Kritz H, Schmid P, Sinzinger H. Passive smoking and cardiovascular risk. *Arch Intern Med*. 1995;155(18):1942-8.

7 Critchley JA, Capewell S. Mortality risk reduction associated with smoking cessation in patients with coronary heart disease: a systematic review. *JAMA*. 2003;290(1):86-97.

8 Law M, Tang JL. An analysis of the effectiveness of interventions intended to help people stop smoking. *Arch Intern Med*. 1995;155(18):1933-41.

9 Ip S, Lichtenstein AH, Chung M, et al. Systematic review: association of low-density lipoprotein subfractions with cardiovascular outcomes. *Ann Intern Med*. 2009 Apr 7;150(7):474-84.

10 Davidson MH. Apolipoprotein measurements: is more widespread use clinically indicated? *Clin Cardiol*. 2009 Sep;32(9):482-6.

11 Centers for Disease Control and Prevention. Trends in leisure-time physical inactivity by age, sex, and race/ethnicity – United States, 1994-2004. *MMWR Morb Mortal Wkly Rep*. 2005 Oct 7;54(39):991-4.

12   Ridker PM, Rifai N, Rose L, et al. Comparison of C-reactive protein and low-density lipoprotein cholesterol levels in the prediction of first cardiovascular events. *N Engl J Med.* 2002;347(20):1557-65.

13   Lee WY, Park JS, Noh SY, et al. C-reactive protein concentrations are related to insulin resistance and metabolic syndrome as defined by the ATP III report. *Int J Cardiol.* 2004;97(1):101-6.

14   Sermet A, Aybak M, Ulak G, et al. Effect of oral pyridoxine hydrochloride supplementation on in vitro platelet sensitivity to different agonists. *Arzneimittelforschung.* 1995;45(1):19-21.

15   Friso S, Girelli D, Martinelli N, et al. Low plasma vitamin B-6 concentrations and modulation of coronary artery disease risk. *Am J Clin Nutr.* 2004;79(6):992-8.

16   Church TS, Earnest CP, Wood KA, et al. Reduction of C-reactive protein levels through use of a multivitamin. *Am J Med.* 2003;115(9):702-7.

17   Kiesewetter H, Jung F, Pindur G, et al. Effect of garlic on thrombocyte aggregation, microcirculation, and other risk factors. *Int J Clin Pharmacol Ther Toxicol.* 1991;29(4):151-5.

18   Ernst E. Fibrinogen: an important risk factor for atherothrombotic diseases. *Ann Med.* 1994;26(1): 15-22.

19   Chrysohoou C, Panagiotakos DB, Pitsavos C, et al. Adherence to the Mediterranean diet attenuates inflammation and coagulation process in healthy adults: the ATTICA Study. *J Am Coll Cardiol.* 2004;44(1):152-8.

20   Hsia CH, Shen MC, Lin JS, et al. Nattokinase decreases plasma levels of fibrinogen, factor VII, and factor VIII in human subjects. *Nutr Res.* 2009 Mar;29(3):190-6.

21   Kim JY, Lee JH, Paik JK, et al. Effects of nattokinase on blood pressure: a randomized, controlled trial. *Hypertens Res.* 2008;31(8):1583-8.

22   Boushey C, Beresford S, Omenn G, et al. A quantitative assessment of plasma homocysteine as a risk factor for vascular disease. Probable benefits of increasing folic acid intakes. *JAMA.* 1995; 274(13):1049-57.

23   Gauthier GM, Keevil JG, McBride PE. The association of homocysteine and coronary artery disease. *Clin Cardiol.* 2003;26(12):563-8.

24   Bozkurt E, Keles S, Acikel M, et al. Plasma homocysteine level and the angiographic extent of coronary artery disease. *Angiology.* 2004;55(3):265-70.

25   Humphrey LL, Fu R, Rogers K, et al. Homocysteine level and CHD incidence: a systematic review and meta-analysis. *Mayo Clin Proc.* 2008 Nov;83(11):1203-12.

26   Ubbink JB, Vermaak WJ, van der Merwe A, et al. Vitamin B-12, vitamin B-6, and folate nutritional status in men with hyperhomocysteinemia. *Am J Clin Nutr.* 1993;57(1):47-53.

27   Anderson JL, Jensen KR, Carlquist JF, et al. Effect of folic acid fortification of food on homocysteine-related mortality. *Am J Med.* 2004;116(3):158-64.

28   Matthews KA, Haynes SG. Type A behavior pattern and coronary disease risk. Update and critical evaluation. *Am J Epidemiol.* 1986;123(6):923-60.

29   Muller MM, Rau H, Brody S. The relationship between habitual anger coping style and serum lipid and lipoprotein concentrations. *Biol Psychol.* 1995;41(1):69-81.

30   Strike PC, Steptoe A. Psychosocial factors in the development of coronary artery disease. *Prog Cardiovasc Dis.* 2004;46(4):337-47.

31   Suarez EC. C-reactive protein is associated with psychological risk factors of cardiovascular disease in apparently healthy adults. *Psychosom Med.* 2004;66(5):684-91.

32   Ornish D, Brown SE, Scherwitz LW, et al. Can lifestyle changes reverse coronary heart disease? The Lifestyle Heart Trial. Lancet. 1990;336(8708):129-33.

33   Burr ML, Fehily AM, Gilbert JF, et al. Effects of changes in fat, fish, and fiber intakes on death and myocardial reinfarction. Diet and Reinfarction Trial (DART). Lancet. 1989;2(8666):757-61.

34   de Lorgeril M, Renaud S, Mamelle N, et al. Mediterranean alpha-linolenic acid-rich diet in secondary prevention of coronary heart disease. Lancet. 1994;343(8911):1454-9.

35   Weil J, Colin-Jones D, Langman M, et al. Prophylactic aspirin and risk of peptic ulcer bleeding. BMJ. 1995;310(6983):827-30.

CHAPTER 2 - BASIC DIETARY AND SUPPLEMENT STRATEGIES FOR HEART HEALTH

1   Sieri S, Krogh V, Berrino F, et al. Dietary glycemic load and index and risk of coronary heart disease in a large Italian cohort: the EPICOR study. Arch Intern Med. 2010 Apr 12;170(7):640-7.

2   Esposito K, Marfella R, Ciotola M, et al. Effect of a Mediterranean-style diet on endothelial dysfunction and markers of vascular inflammation in the metabolic syndrome: a randomized trial. JAMA. 2004;292(12):1440-6.

3   Martinez-Gonzalez MA, Sanchez-Villegas A. The emerging role of Mediterranean diets in cardiovascular epidemiology: monounsaturated fats, olive oil, red wine or the whole pattern? Eur J Epidemiol. 2004;19(1):9-13.

4   Alarcon de la Lastra C, Barranco MD, Motilva V, et al. Mediterranean diet and health: biological importance of olive oil. Curr Pharm Des. 2001;7:933-50.

5   Bucher HC, Hengstler P, Schindler C, et al. N-3 polyunsaturated fatty acids in coronary heart disease: a meta-analysis of randomized controlled trials. Am J Med. 2002;112:298-304.

6   Harris WS, Von Schacky C. The Omega-3 Index: a new risk factor for death from coronary heart disease? Prev Med. 2004;39(1):212-20.

7   Harris WS. The omega-3 index as a risk factor for coronary heart disease. Am J Clin Nutr. 2008 Jun;87(6):1997S-2002S.

8   Hu FB, Bronner L, Willett WC, et al. Fish and omega-3 fatty acid intake and risk of coronary heart disease in women. JAMA. 2002;287(14):1815-21.

9   Albert CM, Campos H, Stampfer MJ, et al. Blood levels of long-chain n-3 fatty acids and the risk of sudden death. N Engl J Med. 2002;346(15):1113-8.

10   Skulas-Ray AC, Kris-Etherton PM, Harris WS, et al. Dose-response effects of omega-3 fatty acids on triglycerides, inflammation, and endothelial function in healthy persons with moderate hypertriglyceridemia. Am J Clin Nutr. 2011 Feb;93(2):243-52.

11   Sandker GW, Kromhout D, Aravanis C, et al. Serum cholesterol ester fatty acids and their relation with serum lipids in elderly men in Crete and the Netherlands. Eur J Clin Nutr. 1993;47(3):201-8.

12   Kagawa Y, Nishizawa M, Suzuki M, et al. Eicosapolyenoic acids of serum lipids of Japanese Islanders with low incidence of cardiovascular diseases. J Nutr Sci Vitaminol (Tokyo). 1982;28(4):441-53.

13   Hu FB, Stampfer MJ. Nut consumption and risk of coronary heart disease: a review of epidemiologic evidence. Curr Atheroscler Rep. 1999;1(3):204-9.

14   Ros E, Nunez I, Perez-Heras A, et al. A walnut diet improves endothelial function in hypercholesterolemic subjects: a randomized crossover trial. Circulation. 2004;109(13):1609-14.

15   Ford ES, Liu S, Mannino DM, et al. C-reactive protein concentration and concentrations of blood vitamins, carotenoids, and selenium among United States adults. *Eur J Clin Nutr.* 2003;57(9): 1157-63.

16   Floegel A, Chung SJ, von Ruesten A, et al. Antioxidant intake from diet and supplements and elevated serum C-reactive protein and plasma homocysteine concentrations in US adults: a cross-sectional study. *Public Health Nutr.* 2011 Nov;14(11):2055-64.

17   Weisburger JH. Lycopene and tomato products in health promotion. *Exp Biol Med.* 2002; 227(10): 924-7.

18   Williams MJ, Sutherland WH, Whelan AP, et al. Acute effect of drinking red and white wines on circulating levels of inflammation-sensitive molecules in men with coronary artery disease. *Metabolism.* 2004;53(3):318-23.

19   Rimm EB, Williams P, Fosher K, et al. Moderate alcohol intake and lower risk of coronary heart disease: meta-analysis of effects on lipids and haemostatic factors. *BMJ.* 1999;319(7224):1523-8.

20   Lekakis J, Rallidis LS, Andreadou I, et al. Polyphenolic compounds from red grapes acutely improve endothelial function in patients with coronary heart disease. *Eur J Cardiovasc Prev Rehabil.* 2005;12(6):596-600.

21   Oak MH, El Bedoui J, Schini-Kerth VB. Antiangiogenic properties of natural polyphenols from red wine and green tea. *J Nutr Biochem.* 2005;16(1):1-8.

22   Sumner MD, Elliott-Eller M, Weidner G, et al. Effects of pomegranate juice consumption on myocardial perfusion in patients with coronary heart disease. *Am J Cardiol.* 2005;96(6):810-4.

23   Aviram M, Rosenblat M, Gaitini D, et al. Pomegranate juice consumption for 3 years by patients with carotid artery stenosis reduces common carotid intima-media thickness, blood pressure and LDL oxidation. *Clin Nutr.* 2004;23(3):423-33.

24   Esmaillzadeh A, Tahbaz F, Gaieni I, et al. Concentrated pomegranate juice improves lipid profiles in diabetic patients with hyperlipidemia. *J Med Food.* 2004;7(3):305-8.

25   Whelton PK, He J. Potassium in preventing and treating high blood pressure. *Semin Nephrol.* 1999;19(5):494-9.

26   Sacks FM, Svetkey LP, Vollmer WM, et al. Effects on blood pressure of reduced dietary sodium and the Dietary Approaches to Stop Hypertension (DASH) diet. DASH–Sodium Collaborative Research Group. *N Engl J Med.* 2001;344(1):3-10.

27   Jansson B. Potassium, sodium, and cancer: a review. *J Env Pathol Toxicol Oncol.* 1996;15(2-4):65-73.

28   Maier JA. Low magnesium and atherosclerosis: an evidence-based link. *Mol Aspects Med.* 2003;24 (1-3):137-46.

29   Maier JA, Malpuech-Brugere C, Zimowska W, et al. Low magnesium promotes endothelial cell dysfunction: implications for atherosclerosis, inflammation and thrombosis. *Biochim Biophys Acta.* 2004;1689(1):13-21.

30   Clarke R, Armitage J. Antioxidant vitamins and risk of cardiovascular disease. Review of large-scale randomised trials. *Cardiovasc Drugs Ther.* 2002;16(5):411-5.

31   Vivekananthan DP, Penn MS, Sapp SK, et al. Use of antioxidant vitamins for the prevention of cardiovascular disease: meta-analysis of randomised trials. *Lancet.* 2003;361(9374):2017-23.

32   Salonen RM, Nyyssonen K, Kaikkonen J, et al. Six-year effect of combined vitamin C and E supplementation on atherosclerotic progression: the Antioxidant Supplementation in Atherosclerosis Prevention (ASAP) Study. *Circulation.* 2003;107(7):947-53.

33   Saremi A, Arora R. Vitamin E and cardiovascular disease. *Am J Ther.* 2010 May-Jun;17(3):e56-65.

34   Yegin A, Yegin H, Aliciguzel Y, et al. Erythrocyte selenium-glutathione peroxidase activity is lower in patients with coronary atherosclerosis. *Jpn Heart J.* 1997;38(6):793-8.

35   Simon JA. Vitamin C and cardiovascular disease: a review. *J Am Coll Nutr.* 1992;11(2):107-25.

36   Harats D, Ben-Naim M, Dabach Y, et al. Effect of vitamin C and E supplementation on susceptibility of plasma lipoproteins to peroxidation induced by acute smoking. *Atherosclerosis.* 1990;85(1): 47-54.

37   Hallfrisch J, Singh VN, Muller DC, et al. High plasma vitamin C associated with high plasma HDL- and HDL2 cholesterol. *Am J Clin Nutr.* 1994;60(1):100-5.

38   Kim DH, Sabour S, Sagar UN, et al. Prevalence of hypovitaminosis D in cardiovascular diseases (from the National Health and Nutrition Examination Survey 2001 to 2004). *Am J Cardiol.* 2008 Dec 1;102(11):1540-4.

39   Dobnig H, Pilz S, Scharnagl H, et al. Independent association of low serum 25-hydroxyvitamin d and 1,25-dihydroxyvitamin d levels with all-cause and cardiovascular mortality. *Arch Intern Med.* 2008 Jun 23;168(12):1340-9.

CHAPTER 3 – THE TRUTH ABOUT STATINS, CHOLESTEROL, AND NATURAL ALTERNATIVES

1   Ip S, Lichtenstein AH, Chung M, et al. Systematic review: association of low-density lipoprotein subfractions with cardiovascular outcomes. *Ann Intern Med.* 2009 Apr 7;150(7):474-84.

2   Davidson MH. Apolipoprotein measurements: is more widespread use clinically indicated? *Clin Cardiol.* 2009 Sep;32(9):482-6.

3   Schaefer EJ, Lamon-Fava S, Jenner JL, et al. Lipoprotein(a) levels and risk of coronary heart disease in men. The Lipid Research Clinics Coronary Primary Prevention Trial. *JAMA.* 1994;271(13): 999-1003.

4   Kannel WB, Vasan RS. Triglycerides as vascular risk factors: new epidemiologic insights. *Curr Opin Cardiol.* 2009 Jul;24(4):345-50.

5   Stalenhoef AF, de Graaf J. Association of fasting and nonfasting serum triglycerides with cardiovascular disease and the role of remnant-like lipoproteins and small dense LDL. *Curr Opin Lipidol.* 2008 Aug;19(4):355-61.

6   Culver AL, Ockene IS, Balasubramanian R, et al. Statin use and risk of diabetes mellitus in postmenopausal women in the Women's Health Initiative. *Arch Intern Med.* 2012 Jan 23;172(2):144-52.

7   Heart Protection Study Collaborative Group. MRC/BHF Heart Protection Study of cholesterol lowering with simvastatin in 20,536 high-risk individuals: a randomised placebo-controlled trial. *Lancet.* 2002;360(9326):7-22.

8   Thavendiranathan P, Bagai A, Brookhart MA, et al. Primary prevention of cardiovascular diseases with statin therapy: a meta-analysis of randomized controlled trials. *Arch Intern Med.* 2006 Nov 27; 166(21):2307-13.

9   Baigent C, Keech A, Kearney PM, et al. Cholesterol Treatment Trialists' Collaborators. Efficacy and safety of cholesterol-lowering treatment: prospective meta-analysis of data from 90 056 participants in 14 randomised trials of statins. *Lancet.* 2005;366(9493):1267-78.

10   Vrecer M, Turk S, Drinovec J, et al. Use of statins in primary and secondary prevention of coronary heart disease and ischemic stroke. Meta-analysis of randomized trials. *Int J Clin Pharmacol Ther*. 2003;41(12):567-77.

11   Ray KK, Seshasai SR, Erqou S, et al. Statins and all-cause mortality in high-risk primary prevention: a meta-analysis of 11 randomized controlled trials involving 65,229 participants. *Arch Intern Med*. 2010 Jun 28;170(12):1024-31.

12   Hakim AA, Petrovitch H, Burchfiel CM, et al. Effects of walking on mortality among nonsmoking retired men. *N Engl J Med*. 1998;338(2):94-9.

13   Naska A, Oikonomou E, Trichopoulou A, et al. Siesta in healthy adults and coronary mortality in the general population. *Arch Intern Med*. 2007;167(3):296-301.

14   Littarru GP, Langsjoen P. Coenzyme Q_{10} and statins: biochemical and clinical implications. *Mitochondrion*. 2007;7(Suppl.):S168-74.

15   Walsh JME, Pignone M. Drug treatment of hyperlipidemia in women. *JAMA*. 204;291(18): 2243-52.

16   Shepherd J, Blauw GJ, Murphy MB, et al. Pravastatin in elderly individuals at risk of vascular disease (PROSPER): a randomised controlled trial. *Lancet*. 2002;360(9346):1623-30.

17   ALLHAT Officers and Coordinators for the ALLHAT Collaborative Research Group. The Antihypertensive and Lipid-Lowering Treatment to Prevent Heart Attack Trial. Major outcomes in moderately hypercholesterolemic, hypertensive patients randomized to pravastatin vs usual care. *JAMA*. 2002;288(23):2998-3007.

18   Nakaya N, Kita T, Mabuchi H, et al. Large-scale cohort study on the relationship between serum lipid concentrations and risk of cerebrovascular disease under low-dose simvastatin in Japanese patients with hypercholesterolemia: sub-analysis of the Japan Lipid Intervention Trial (J-LIT). *Circ J*. 2005;69(9):1016-21.

19   Hecht HS, Harman SM. Relation of aggressiveness of lipid-lowering treatment to changes in calcified plaque burden by electron beam tomography. *Am J Cardiol*. 2003;92(3):334-6.

20   Jenkins DJ, Kendall CW, Marchie A, et al. Effects of a dietary portfolio of cholesterol-lowering foods vs lovastatin on serum lipids and C-reactive protein. *JAMA*. 2003;290(4):502-10.

21   Jenkins DJ, Kendall CW, Faulkner DA, et al. Long-term effects of a plant-based dietary portfolio of cholesterol-lowering foods on blood pressure. *Eur J Clin Nutr*. 2008 Jun;62(6):781-8.

22   Gigleux I, Jenkins DJ, Kendall CW, et al. Comparison of a dietary portfolio diet of cholesterol-lowering foods and a statin on LDL particle size phenotype in hypercholesterolaemic participants. *Br J Nutr*. 2007 Dec;98(6):1229-36.

23   Reynolds K, Chin A, Lees KA, et al. A meta-analysis of the effect of soy protein supplementation on serum lipids. *Am J Cardiol*. 2006;98(5):633-40.

24   Anderson JW, Johnstone BM, Cook-Newell ME. Meta-analysis of the effects of soy protein intake on serum lipids. *N Engl J Med*. 1995;333(5):276-82.

25   Langsjoen PH, Langsjoen AM. The clinical use of HMG CoA-reductase inhibitors and the associated depletion of coenzyme Q_{10}. A review of animal and human publications. *Biofactors*. 2003;18(1-4):101-11.

26   Rundek T, Naini A, Sacco R, et al. Atorvastatin decreases the coenzyme Q_{10} level in the blood of patients at risk for cardiovascular disease and stroke. *Arch Neurol*. 2004;61(6):889-92.

27   McNamara DJ. Dietary cholesterol and atherosclerosis. *Biochim Biophys Acta*. 2000 Dec 15; 1529 (1-3):310-20.

28 Glore SR, Van Treeck D, Knehans AW, Guild M. Soluble fiber and serum lipids: a literature review. *J Am Diet Assoc.* 1994;94(4):425-36.

29 Lyon MR, Reichert RG. The effect of a novel polysaccharide along with lifestyle changes on short-term weight loss and associated risk factors in overweight and obese adults: an observational retrospective clinical analysis. *Altern Med Rev.* 2010;15(1):68-75.

30 Lyon M, Wood S, Pelletier X, et al. Effects of a 3-month supplementation with a novel soluble highly viscous polysaccharide on anthropometry and blood lipids in nondieting overweight or obese adults. *J Hum Nutr Diet.* 2011 Aug;24(4):351-9. doi: 10.1111/j.1365-277X.2011.01157.x.

31 Ripsin CM, Keenan JM, Jacobs DR, et al. Oat products and lipid lowering, a meta-analysis. *JAMA.* 1992;267(24):3317-25.

32 Ajani UA, Ford ES, Mokdad AH. Dietary fiber and C-reactive protein: findings from national health and nutrition examination survey data. *J Nutr.* 2004;134(5):1181-5.

33 Weitz D, Weintraub H, Fisher E, et al. Fish oil for the treatment of cardiovascular disease. *Cardiol Rev.* 2010 Sep-Oct;18(5):258-63.

34 McKenney JM, Sica D. Role of prescription omega-3 fatty acids in the treatment of hypertriglyceridemia. *Pharmacotherapy.* 2007 May;27(5):715-28.

35 Musa-Veloso K, Binns MA, Kocenas AC, et al. Long-chain omega-3 fatty acids eicosapentaenoic acid and docosahexaenoic acid dose-dependently reduce fasting serum triglycerides. *Nutr Rev.* 2010 Mar;68(3):155-67.

36 Skulas-Ray AC, Kris-Etherton PM, Harris WS, et al. Dose-response effects of omega-3 fatty acids on triglycerides, inflammation, and endothelial function in healthy persons with moderate hypertriglyceridemia. *Am J Clin Nutr.* 2011 Feb;93(2):243-52.

37 Davidson MH. Mechanisms for the hypotriglyceridemic effect of marine omega-3 fatty acids. *Am J Cardiol.* 2006 Aug 21;98(4A):27i-33i.

38 Canner PL, Berge KG, Wenger NK, et al. Fifteen year mortality in Coronary Drug Project patients: long-term benefit with niacin. *J Am Coll Cardiol.* 1986;8(6):1245-55.

39 DiPalma JR, Thayer WS. Use of niacin as a drug. *Annu Rev Nutr.* 1991;11:169-87.

40 Illingworth DR, Stein EA, Mitchel YB, et al. Comparative effects of lovastatin and niacin in primary hypercholesterolemia. A prospective trial. *Arch Intern Med.* 1994;154(14):1586-95.

41 Carlson LA, Hamsten A, Asplund A. Pronounced lowering of serum levels of lipoprotein Lp(a) in hyperlipidaemic subjects treated with nicotinic acid. *J Intern Med.* 1989;226(4):271-6.

42 Pan J, Lin M, Kesala RL, et al. Niacin treatment of the atherogenic lipid profile and Lp(a) in diabetes. *Diabetes Obes Metab.* 2002;4(4):255-61.

43 Vega GL, Grundy SM. Lipoprotein responses to treatment with lovastatin, gemfibrozil, and nicotinic acid in normolipidemic patients with hypoalphalipoproteinemia. *Arch Intern Med.* 1994; 154(1):73-82.

44 Van JT, Pan J, Wasty T, et al. Comparison of extended-release niacin and atorvastatin monotherapies and combination treatment of the atherogenic lipid profile in diabetes mellitus. *Am J Cardiol.* 2002; 89(11):1306-8.

45 Rindone JP, Achacoso S. Effect of low-dose niacin on glucose control in patients with non–insulin-dependent diabetes mellitus and hyperlipidemia. *Am J Ther.* 1996;3(9):637-9.

46 Kane MP, Hamilton RA, Addesse E, et al. Cholesterol and glycemic effects of Niaspan in patients with type 2 diabetes. *Pharmacotherapy.* 2001;21(12):1473-8.

47   Kuvin JT, Dave DM, Sliney KA, et al. Effects of extended-release niacin on lipoprotein particle size, distribution, and inflammatory markers in patients with coronary artery disease. *Am J Cardiol.* 2006;98(6):743-5.

48   McKenney JM, Proctor JD, Harris S, et al. A comparison of the efficacy and toxic effects of sustained- vs immediate-release niacin in hypercholesterolemic patients. *JAMA.* 1994; 271(9):672-7.

49   Goldberg AC. A meta-analysis of randomized controlled studies on the effects of extended-release niacin in women. *Am J Cardiol.* 2004;94(1):121-4.

50   Guyton JR. Extended-release niacin for modifying the lipoprotein profile. *Expert Opin Pharmacother.* 2004;5(6):1385-98.

51   Rubenfire M. Impact of Medical Subspecialty on Patient Compliance to Treatment Study Group. Safety and compliance with once-daily niacin extended-release/lovastatin as initial therapy in the Impact of Medical Subspecialty on Patient Compliance to Treatment (IMPACT) study. *Am J Cardiol.* 2004;94(3):306-11.

52   Vogt A, Kassner U, Hostalek U, et al. NAUTILUS Study Group. Evaluation of the safety and tolerability of prolonged-release nicotinic acid in a usual care setting: the NAUTILUS study. *Curr Med Res Opin.* 2006;22(2):417-25.

53   Welsh AL, Ede M. Inositol hexanicotinate for improved nicotinic acid therapy. Preliminary report. *Int Rec Med.* 1961;174:9-15.

54   El-Enein AMA, Hafez YS, Salem H, et al. The role of nicotinic acid and inositol hexaniacinate as anticholesterolemic and antilipemic agents. *Nutr Rep Int.* 1983;28:899-911.

55   Roza JM, Xian-Liu Z, Guthrie N. Effect of citrus flavonoids and tocotrienols on serum cholesterol levels in hypercholesterolemic subjects. *Altern Ther Health.* Med 2007;13(6):44-8.

56   Ostlund RE Jr. Phytosterols and cholesterol metabolism. *Curr Opin Lipidol.* 2004;15(1):37-41.

57   Miettinen TA, Gylling H. Plant stanol and sterol esters in prevention of cardiovascular diseases. *Ann Med.* 2004;36(2):126-34.

58   Kozlowska-Wojciechowska M, Jastrzebska M, Naruszewicz M, et al. Impact of margarine enriched with plant sterols on blood lipids, platelet function, and fibrinogen level in young men. *Metabolism.* 2003;52(11):1373-8.

59   Yoshida Y, Niki E. Antioxidant effects of phytosterol and its components. *J Nutr Sci Vitaminol* (Tokyo). 2003;49(4):277-80.

60   de Jong A, Plat J, Mensink RP. Metabolic effects of plant sterols and stanols (review). *J Nutr Biochem.* 2003;14(7):362-9.

61   Arsenio L, Bodria P, Magnati G, et al. Effectiveness of long-term treatment with pantethine in patients with dyslipidemias. *Clin Ther.* 1986;8(5):537-45.

62   Gaddi A, Descovich GC, Noseda P, et al. Controlled evaluation of pantethine, a natural hypolipidemic compound, in patients with different forms of hyperlipoproteinemia. *Atherosclerosis.* 1984;50(1):73-83.

63   Coronel F, Tomero F, Torrente J, et al. Treatment of hyperlipemia in diabetic patients on dialysis with a physiological substance. *Am J Nephrol.* 1991;11(1):32-6.

64   Donati C, Bertieri RS, Barbi G. [Pantethine, diabetes mellitus and atherosclerosis. Clinical study of 1045 patients]. *Clin Ter.* 1989;128(6):411-22.

65   Hiramatsu K, Nozaki H, Arimori S. Influence of pantethine on platelet volume, microviscosity, lipid composition and functions in diabetes mellitus with hyperlipidemia. *Tokai J Exp Clin Med.* 1981;6(1):49-57.

66 Lawson LD, Wang ZJ, Papdimitrou D. Allicin release under simulated gastrointestinal conditions from garlic powder tablets employed in clinical trials on serum cholesterol. *Planta Med.* 2001; 67(1):13-8.

67 Lawson LD, Wang ZJ. Tablet quality: a major problem in clinical trials with garlic supplements. *Forsch Komplementmed.* 2000;7:45.

68 Banerjee SK, Maulik SK. Effect of garlic on cardiovascular disorders: a review. *Nutr J.* 2002;1:4.

69 Alder R, Lookinland S, Berry JA, et al. A systematic review of the effectiveness of garlic as an anti-hyperlipidemic agent. *J Am Acad Nurse Pract.* 2003;15(3):120-9.

70 Stevinson C, Pittler MH, Erst E. Garlic for treating hypercholesterolemia. A meta-analysis of randomized clinical trials. *Ann Intern Med.* 2000;133(6):420-9.

CHAPTER 4 - BEYOND CHOLESTEROL: THE ROLE OF INSULIN RESISTANCE

1 Jia H, Lubetkin EI. Trends in quality-adjusted life-years lost contributed by smoking and obesity. *Am J Prev Med.* 2010 Feb;38(2):138-44.

2 Jia H, Lubetkin EI. Obesity-related quality-adjusted life years lost in the U.S. from 1993 to 2008. *Am J Prev Med.* 2010 Sep;39(3):220-7.

3 Finkelstein EA, Trogdon JG, Cohen JW, et al. Annual medical spending attributable to obesity: payer- and service-specific estimates. *Health Aff (Millwood).* 2009;28(5):w822-31.

4 Yamagishi SI, Nakamura K, Matsui T, et al. Role of postprandial hyperglycaemia in cardiovascular disease in diabetes. *Int J Clin Pract.* 2007 Jan;61(1):83-7.

5 Blaak EE, Antoine JM, Benton D, et al. Impact of postprandial glycaemia on health and prevention of disease. *Obes Rev.* 2012 Oct;13(10):923-84.

6 Wursch P, Pi-Sunyer FX. The role of viscous soluble fiber in the metabolic control of diabetes. A review with special emphasis on cereals rich in beta-glucan. *Diabetes Care.* 1997;20(11):1774-80.

7 Slama G. Dietary therapy in type 2 diabetes oriented towards postprandial blood glucose improvement. *Diabetes Metab Rev.* 1998;14(Suppl 1):S19-24.

8 Montonen J, Knekt P, Jarvinen R, et al. Whole-grain and fiber intake and the incidence of type 2 diabetes. *Am J Clin Nutr.* 2003;77(3):622-9.

9 Fung TT, Hu FB, Pereira MA, et al. Whole-grain intake and the risk of type 2 diabetes: a prospective study in men. *Am J Clin Nutr.* 2002;76(3):535-40.

10 Brand-Miller JC, Atkinson FS, Gahler RJ, et al. Effects of PGX, a novel functional fibre, on acute and delayed postprandial glycaemia. *Eur J Clin Nutr.* 2010 Dec;64(12):1488-93.

11 Brand-Miller JC, Atkinson FS, Gahler RJ, et al. Effects of added PGX*, a novel functional fibre, on the glycaemic index of starchy foods. *Br J Nutr.* 2012 Jul;108(2):245-8.

12 Jenkins AL, Kacinik V, Lyon MR, et al. Reduction of postprandial glycemia by the novel viscous polysaccharide PGX, in a dose-dependent manner, independent of food form. *J Am Coll Nutr.* 2010 Apr;29(2):92-8.

13 Hung T, Sievenpiper JL, Marchie A, et al. Fat versus carbohydrate in insulin resistance, obesity, diabetes and cardiovascular disease. *Curr Opin Clin Nutr Metab Care.* 2003;6(2):165-76.

14 Salmeron J, Hu FB, Manson JE, et al. Dietary fat intake and risk of type 2 diabetes in women. *Am J Clin Nutr.* 2001;73(6):1019-26.

15 Rivellese AA, De Natale C, Lilli S. Type of dietary fat and insulin resistance. *Ann N Y Acad Sci.* 2002;967:329-35.

16 Jiang R, Manson JE, Stampfer MJ, et al. Nut and peanut butter consumption and risk of type 2 diabetes in women. *JAMA.* 2002;288(20):2554-60.

17 Reimer RA, Pelletier X, Carabin IG, et al. Increased plasma PYY levels following supplementation with the functional fiber PolyGlycopleX in healthy adults. *Eur J Clin Nutr.* 2010 Oct;64(10): 1186-91.

18 Lyon MR, Reichert RG. The effect of a novel viscous polysaccharide along with lifestyle changes on short-term weight loss and associated risk factors in overweight and obese adults: an observational retrospective clinical program analysis. *Altern Med Rev.* 2010 Apr;15(1):68-75.

CHAPTER 5 - THE HEART HEALTHY LIFESTYLE

1 Muller MM, Rau H, Brody S, et al. The relationship between habitual anger coping style and serum lipid and lipoprotein concentrations. *Biol Psychol.* 1995;41(1):69-81.

2 Strike PC, Steptoe A. Psychosocial factors in the development of coronary artery disease. *Prog Cardiovasc Dis.* 2004;46(4):337-47.

3 Suarez EC. C-reactive protein is associated with psychological risk factors of cardiovascular disease in apparently healthy adults. *Psychosom Med.* 2004;66(5):684-91.

4 Benson H. The relaxation response: therapeutic effect. *Science.* 1997;278(5344):1694-51.

5 Blair SN, Kohl HW 3rd, Barlow CE, et al. Changes in physical fitness and all-cause mortality. A prospective study of healthy and unhealthy men. *JAMA.* 1995;273(14):1093-8.

6 Farrell SW, Finley CE, Grundy SM. Cardiorespiratory fitness, LDL cholesterol, and CHD mortality in men. *Med Sci Sports Exerc.* 2012 Nov;44(11):2132-7.

CHAPTER 6 - HIGH BLOOD PRESSURE

1 Fogari R, Zoppi A, Corradi L, et al. Effect of body weight loss and normalization on blood pressure in overweight non-obese patients with stage 1 hypertension. *Hypertens Res.* 2010 Mar;33(3):236-42.

2 Navaneethan SD, Yehnert H, Moustarah F, et al. Weight loss interventions in chronic kidney disease: a systematic review and meta-analysis. *Clin J Am Soc Nephrol.* 2009 Oct;4(10):1565-74.

3 Rouse IL, Beilin LJ, Mahoney DP, et al. Vegetarian diet and blood pressure. *Lancet.* 1983; 2(8352):742-3.

4 John JH, Ziebland S, Yudkin P, et al. Oxford Fruit and Vegetable Study Group. Effects of fruit and vegetable consumption on plasma antioxidant concentrations and blood pressure: a randomised controlled trial. *Lancet.* 2002;359(9322):1969-74.

5 Yasunari K, Maeda K, Nakamura M, et al. Oxidative stress in leukocytes is a possible link between blood pressure, blood glucose, and C-reacting protein. *Hypertension.* 2002;39 (3):777-80.

6 Ortiz MC, Manriquez MC, Romero JC, et al. Antioxidants block angiotensin II-induced increases in blood pressure and endothelin. *Hypertension.* 2001;38(3 Pt 2):655-9.

7 Tsi D, Tan BKH. Cardiovascular pharmacology of 3-n-butylphthalide in spontaneously hypertensive rats. *Phytother Res.* 1997;11:576-82.

8   Silagy CA, Neil HA. A meta-analysis of the effect of garlic on blood pressure. *J Hypertens.* 1994;12(4):463-8.

9   Appel LJ, Moore TJ, Obarzanek E, et al. A clinical trial of the effects of dietary patterns on blood pressure. DASH Collaborative Research Group. *N Engl J Med.* 1997;336(16):1117-24.

10   Moore TJ, Conlin PR, Ard J, et al. DASH (Dietary Approaches to Stop Hypertension) diet is effective treatment for stage 1 isolated systolic hypertension. *Hypertension.* 2001;38(2):155-8.

11   Sacks FM, Svetkey LP, Vollmer WM, et al. Effects on blood pressure of reduced dietary sodium and the Dietary Approaches to Stop Hypertension (DASH) diet. DASH-Sodium Collaborative Research Group. *N Engl J Med.* 2001;344(1):3-10.

12   Fujita H, Yoshikawa M. LKPNM: a prodrug-type ACE-inhibitory peptide derived from fish protein. *Immunopharmacology.* 1999;44(1-2):123-7.

13   Fujita H, Yamagami T, Ohshima K. Effects of an ace-inhibitory agent, katsuobushi oligopeptide, in the spontaneously hypertensive rat and in borderline and mildly hypertensive subjects. *Nutr Res.* 2001;21:1149-58.

14   Fujita H, Yasumoto R, Hasegawa M, et al. Antihypertensive activity of "Katsuobushi Oligopeptide" in hypertensive and borderline hypertensive subjects. *Jpn Pharmacol Ther.* 1997;25:147-51.

15   Fujita H, Yasumoto R, Hasegawa M, et al. Antihypertensive activity of "Katsuobushi Oligopeptide" in hypertensive and borderline hypertensive subjects. *Jpn Pharmacol Ther.* 1997;25:153-7.

16   Kawasaki T, Seki E, Osajima K, et al. Antihypertensive effect of valyl-tyrosine, a short chain peptide derived from sardine muscle hydrolysate, on mild hypertensive subjects. *J Hum Hypertens.* 2000;14(8):519-23.

17   Langsjoen P, Langsjoen P, Willis R, et al. Treatment of essential hypertension with coenzyme Q10. *Mol Aspects Med.* 1994;15(Suppl):S265-72.

18   Ho MJ, Bellusci A, Wright JM. Blood pressure lowering efficacy of coenzyme Q10 for primary hypertension. *Cochrane Database Syst Rev.* 2009 4:CD007435.

19   Scheffler A, Rauwald HW, Kampa B, et al. *Olea europaea* leaf extract exerts L-type Ca(2+) channel antagonistic effects. *J Ethnopharmacol.* 2008 Nov 20;120(2):233-40.

20   Cherif S, Rahal N, Haouala M, et al. A clinical trial of a titrated Olea extract in the treatment of essential arterial hypertension. J Pharm Belg. 1996;51(2):69-71.

21   Perrinjaquet-Moccetti T, Busjahn A, Schmidlin C, et al. Food supplementation with an olive *(Olea europaea L.)* leaf extract reduces blood pressure in borderline hypertensive monozygotic twins. *Phytother Res.* 2008 Sep;22(9):1239-42.

22   Susalit E, Agus N, Effendi I, et al. Olive *(Olea europaea)* leaf extract effective in patients with stage-1 hypertension: comparison with Captopril. *Phytomedicine.* 2011 Feb 15;18(4):251-8.

23   McKay DL, Chen CY, Saltzman E, et al. *Hibiscus sabdariffa L.* tea (tisane) lowers blood pressure in prehypertensive and mildly hypertensive adults. *J Nutr.* 2010 Feb;140(2):298-303.

24   Mozaffari-Khosravi H, Jalali-Khanabadi BA, Afkhami-Ardekani M, et al. The effects of sour tea *(Hibiscus sabdariffa)* on hypertension in patients with type II diabetes. *J Hum Hypertens.* 2009 Jan;23(1):48-54.

25   Haji Faraji M, Haji Tarkhani A. The effect of sour tea *(Hibiscus sabdariffa)* on essential hypertension. *J Ethnopharmacol.* 1999 Jun;65(3):231-6.

26   Herrera-Arellano A, Miranda-Sánchez J, Avila-Castro P, et al. Clinical effects produced by a standardized herbal medicinal product of *Hibiscus sabdariffa* on patients with hypertension. A randomized, double-blind, lisinopril-controlled clinical trial. *Planta Med.* 2007 Jan;73(1):6-12.

27   Herrera-Arellano A, Flores-Romero S, Chávez-Soto MA, et al. Effectiveness and tolerability of a standardized extract from *Hibiscus sabdariffa* in patients with mild to moderate hypertension: a controlled and randomized clinical trial. *Phytomedicine.* 2004 Jul;11(5):375-82.

CHAPTER 7 – IMPROVING HEART FUNCTION, PLUS SOME SPECIAL CONSIDERATIONS
(ANGIOGRAMS, BYPASS, CHELATION, AND STROKE RECOVERY)

1   Turlapaty PD, Altura BM. Magnesium deficiency produces spasms of coronary arteries: relationship to etiology of sudden death ischemic heart disease. *Science.* 1980;208(4440):198-200.

2   McLean RM. Magnesium and its therapeutic uses: a review. *Am J Med.* 1994;96(1):63-76.

3   Onalan O, Crystal E, Daoulah A, et al. Meta-analysis of magnesium therapy for the acute management of rapid atrial fibrillation. *Am J Cardiol.* 2007 Jun 15;99(12):1726-32.

4   Brodsky MA, Orlov MV, Capparelli EV, et al. Magnesium therapy in new-onset atrial fibrillation. *Am J Cardiol.* 1994 Jun 15;73(16):1227-9.

5   Leslie D, Gheorghiade M. Is there a role for thiamine supplementation in the management of heart failure? *Am Heart J.* 1996;131(6):1248-50.

6   Mendoza CE, Rodriguez F, Rosenberg DG. Reversal of refractory congestive heart failure after thiamine supplementation: report of a case and review of literature. *J Cardiovasc Pharmacol Ther.* 2003;8(4):313-6.

7   Zenuk C, Healey J, Donnelly J, et al. Thiamine deficiency in congestive heart failure patients receiving long term furosemide therapy. *Can J Clin Pharmacol.* 2003;10(4):184-8.

8   Kamikawa T, Suzuki Y, Kobayashi A, et al. Effects of L-carnitine on exercise tolerance in patients with stable angina pectoris. *Jpn Heart J.* 1984;25(4):587-97.

9   Mancini M, Rengo F, Lingetti M, et al. Controlled study on the therapeutic efficacy of propionyl-L-carnitine in patients with congestive heart failure. *Arzneimittelforschung.* 1992;42(9): 1101-4.

10   Pucciarelli G, Matsursi M, Latte S, et al. [The clinical and hemodynamic effects of propionyl-L-carnitine in the treatment of congestive heart failure.] *Clin Ter.* 1992;141(11):379-84.

11   Rizos I. Three-year survival of patients with heart failure caused by dilated cardiomyopathy and L-carnitine administration. *Am Heart J.* 2000;139(2 Pt 3):S120-3.

12   Kamikawa T, Kobayashi A, Yamashita T, et al. Effects of coenzyme Q_{10} on exercise tolerance in chronic stable angina pectoris. *Am J Cardiol.* 1985;56(4):247-51.

13   Baggio E, Gandini R, Plancher AC, et al. Italian multicenter study on the safety and efficacy of coenzyme Q_{10} as adjunctive therapy in heart failure. CoQ_{10} Drug Surveillance Investigators. *Mol Aspects Med.* 1994;15(Suppl):S287-94.

14   Langsjoen PH, Langsjoen AM. Supplemental ubiquinol in patients with advanced congestive heart failure. *Biofactors.* 2008;32(1-4):119-28.

15   Rigelsky JM, Sweet BV. Hawthorn: pharmacology and therapeutic uses. *Am J Health Syst Pharm.* 2002;59(5):417-22.

16   Walker AF, Marakis G, Morris AP, et al. Promising hypotensive effect of hawthorn extract: a randomized double-blind pilot study of mild, essential hypertension. *Phytother Res.* 2002;16(1):48-54.

17   Holubarsch CJ, Colucci WS, Meinertz T, et al. SPICE Trial Study Group. The efficacy and safety of Crataegus extract WS 1442 in patients with heart failure: the SPICE trial. *Eur J Heart Fail.* 2008 Dec;10(12):1255-63.